Here's How to Provide Intervention for Children with Autism Spectrum Disorder

A Balanced Approach

Here's How Series

Thomas Murry, PhD
Series Editor

Here's How to Provide Intervention for Children with Autism Spectrum Disorder

A Balanced Approach

Catherine B. Zenko, MS, CCC-SLP
Michelle Peters Hite, MS, CCC-SLP

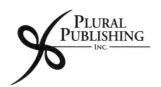

PLURAL
PUBLISHING
INC.

KH

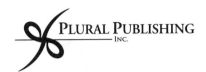

5521 Ruffin Road
San Diego, CA 92123

e-mail: info@pluralpublishing.com
Website: http://www.pluralpublishing.com

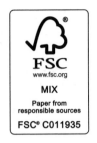

Copyright © by Plural Publishing, Inc. 2014

Typeset in 11/15 Stone Informal by Flanagan's Publishing Services, Inc.
Printed in the United States of America by McNaughton & Gunn, Inc.

Cover photograph © 2013 Maria R. Brea-Spahn

Library of Congress Cataloging-in-Publication Data

Zenko, Catherine B., author.
  Here's how to provide intervention for children with autism spectrum disorder : a balanced
approach / Catherine B. Zenko, Michelle Peters Hite.
      p. ; cm. — (Here's how series)
  Includes bibliographical references and index.
  ISBN-13: 978-1-59756-460-1 (alk. paper)
  ISBN-10: 1-59756-460-5 (alk. paper)
  I. Hite, Michelle Peters, author. II. Title. III. Series: Here's how series.
  [DNLM: 1. Child Development Disorders, Pervasive--therapy. 2. Child. 3. Communication
Disorders—therapy. 4. Early Intervention (Education) 5. Speech-Language Pathology—
methods. WS 350.8.P4]
  RJ506.A9
  618.92'85882—dc23
                                                                    2013019943

9/30/15

Contents

CHAPTER 7 BRINGING IT ALL TOGETHER: APPLICATION AND VIDEO EXAMPLES

147

Foreword

This is the fifth book in the "Here's How" series, a group of texts that focus on a hands-on approach to intervention. This series emanated out of an observation that speech-language pathologists, who work in varied environments, hospitals, clinics, school systems, and private practices, want and need books that go directly to the care of individuals and families. This edition, *Here's How to Provide Intervention for Children with Autism Spectrum Disorder: A Balanced Approach,* by Catherine B. Zenko and Michelle Peters Hite, provides the pathways to understanding the child with autism spectrum disorder (ASD), as well as an insight to the issues underlying the treatments provided by the authors.

The authors have outlined how to design a balanced intervention program for working with children with ASD. They take us on a direct journey to building a balanced intervention program beginning with a comprehensive assessment. They show the clinician how to reach across all levels of social communication using existing evidence and clinical insight. Because speech-language pathologists (SLPs) are involved in the diagnostic process with individuals with ASDs in multiple ways, the authors focus on collaborating within a diagnostic team composed of many medical and/or educational professionals determining whether or not a child has ASD and then implementing an intervention plan that focuses on social communication. Observation of and interaction with the child and their caregivers are integral in the assessment process according to the authors.

Treatment is devoted to a thorough review and descriptions of communication and language skills needed to succeed in an academic setting. The authors integrate the characteristics of ASD, especially the vast cognitive differences in executive function and central coherence, and how they affect all areas of learning. Exceptional in this "Here's How" text are the strategies offered that help improve academic learning and communication. In all, the authors offer solid grounding of their treatments that are based on the underlying cognitive characteristics of ASD and how the SLP fits into the educational process.

Clinicians, both beginning and advanced, will find this book to be a treasure of ideas, clinical insights, and well-documented pathways in the diagnosis and treatment of ASD. They have included the term *balanced intervention* in their title for a reason. This book balances the existing evidence of communication for the child with ASD with maximum *hands-on* treatment approaches. Anyone who has children with ASD on their caseload will want this book close by as a daily partner.

Thomas Murry, PhD
Series Editor

Preface

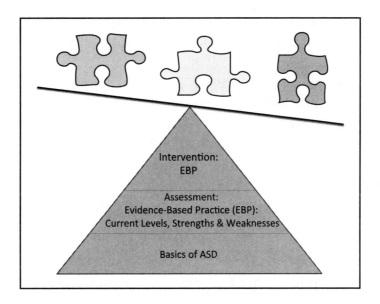

The theme of this book is balance. Autism spectrum disorder (ASD) is a complex disorder that requires careful intervention and educational planning. Through balanced intervention, children with ASD can make strides toward reaching the ultimate goal: successful adult outcomes and independence. What do we mean by balanced intervention? The speech-language pathologist (SLP) must facilitate the design of an intervention plan that will address functional social communication needs, as well as the social communication skills necessary to be successful in the academic environment. The plan should also balance the child's needs across settings: home, school, and community. The SLP works with families, school professionals, community members, and caregivers to determine priorities for intervention and balance all areas targeted. How does the SLP achieve this balance? The graphic above demonstrates the important aspects needed to strike this balance for children with ASD. First, the SLP needs to understand what it means to have ASD. This knowledge serves as the solid foundation that provides the structure and support to achieving balance. Although individuals with ASD are each uniquely different, there are core features that are important to understand. Chapters 1 and 2 give the reader the information needed to understand the key features associated with ASD and how this affects learning, communication, and behavior. Armed with this foundational knowledge, the SLP can then design an assessment that addresses all areas of concern. This assessment then provides the road map for which areas should be targeted within intervention. Chapter 3 provides information on assessing children known to be or suspected of being on the spectrum. Finally, the SLP uses knowledge of evidence-based practice to address the child's core needs within a comprehensive, and balanced, intervention program. This is the ultimate goal for the SLP, and we have devoted three separate chapters to intervention. Chapter 4 provides an overview of evidence-based practices for working with children with ASD. Chapter 5 delves further into methods for improving the wide range of social communication seen in children with ASD. Chapter 6 gives the reader information on how to help the school-age child with ASD achieve communication skills needed to learn and participate in an academic environment. The final chapter contains several case examples and offers the opportunity to see strategies applied to these cases through video snapshots on the accompanying DVD.

The inspiration for the material in this book arose from our clinical experiences, including our work as consultants. We have had the privilege of consulting with many individuals with ASD and their families, as well as professionals in schools and the community working directly with the children. Working with children with ASD is exciting, with new advances occurring frequently; however, this can be challenging for the SLP with a diverse caseload. With ASD on the rise, SLPs in all pediatric settings are sure to encounter children on the spectrum. SLPs do not always receive exposure to ASD in their clinical training programs. For many SLPs in the field, learning about ASD and how best to provide intervention occurs on the job and within continuing education opportunities. We have had the opportunity to work with many schools and clinics to help provide information about ASD and evidence-based practice when working with this population. With these experiences in mind, we created this book to help provide the SLP with an overview and a place to start in terms of finding answers related to providing intervention with children with ASD. There is no "one size fits all" therapy program that works for all children with ASD; however, the SLP armed with knowledge about ASD and evidence-based practices can design effective, individualized intervention plans. By no means is this manual meant to be an exhaustive collection of all information the SLP will need to know to provide therapy to every child on the autism spectrum. Rather, it is our hope that this text helps point the SLP in the right direction toward research and materials that will answer their clinical questions.

Acknowledgments

There are several people I need to thank who made this book a reality. First, Dr. Christine Sapienza, Associate Dean of the College of Health Sciences and Program Director–Speech Pathology at Jacksonville University, planted the seed of me writing the autism book for Plural's *Here's How* series. At the time, I was in the middle of coauthoring a revision of *Understanding the Nature of Autism, Third Edition,* and told the Plural editor that I was flattered but would not have time to think about another book for a while. Lucky for me, the *Here's How* series was just starting to add new topics to the original work, and Plural was in no rush. Thank you, Plural for waiting for me and giving me this opportunity.

One of the lessons I took away from my first foray into writing was that the process takes five times as long as I initially estimated, and I knew I did not want to do this project alone. The first person that came to mind was Michelle Hite, and it was the best decision I could have made, especially since we share the same intellectual "parents" from the University of South Florida. It helps to have a coauthor who can finish my sentences or who's writing style is so similar that it is hard to tell who wrote what part of each chapter. Thank you, Michelle for making this adventure full of intellectual soul food and laughter!

I would like to thank two of my main professors at University of South Florida who left an indelible impression. Thank you, Dr. Elaine Silliman for taking me under your wing and gently pushing (or nudging) me to go the distance, do the research, and write the thesis that was eventually published. She never let me take the easy way out, and I am forever grateful for her tutelage. I would also like to thank Dr. Sylvia Diehl who shared her love of children with autism with me my first semester of graduate school. Her passion and critical clinical thinking skills stuck with me over all of these years, and she continues to be one of my most cherished colleagues.

The best teachers I have had are the individuals on the autism spectrum whom I have had the privilege to work with and get to know. Each person with autism spectrum disorder has taught me invaluable lessons that help me become a better clinician every day. I would also like to thank all of the families who have welcomed me into their homes and community and shared their children or adults with me. I am and have always been a firm believer that quality intervention involves the entire family, not just the patient or client, and I cherish all of the lessons I have learned from working with each and every family. I would like to extend a special thank you to the families who opened their homes to my graduate students and allowed them to learn from you and your children. To all of the families who agreed to let my students record their time with your children for the purposes of teaching others, you are the ones who made Chapter 7 in this book and the supplemental DVD possible.

To all of my University of Florida students whom I have had the pleasure to teach, thank you for your enthusiasm and desire to learn and for helping me become the teacher I am today. Each year I look forward to the lessons you teach me, the questions you ask, and sharing my knowledge with you.

Finally, I need to thank my family. Mom and dad, thank you for always providing a loving and caring atmosphere and for expecting greatness from all six of us. Your efforts have paid off in spades, and I hope I can do the same for my children. To my boys, Tyler and Spencer, I love you with all my heart, and I want to thank you for your patience with me while I was writing. You both bring me so much joy and make me laugh and smile every single day. Last but not least, I want to thank my dear husband, Frank, for taking on the duties of mom and dad each and every weekend I had to go write. I could not have done this without your help. I promise to take a very long break before I consider my next writing project!

—Catherine B. Zenko, MS, CCC-SLP

To my coauthor and intellectual partner, Cathy, collaborating on this book has been fulfilling, and I would not have wanted to share this journey with anyone else. Even through all of the curveballs life threw at us during this time, we still accomplished our goal and shared some memories I will always remember. I truly could never have done it without you.

I dedicate this book to my grandfather, Blaine Peters, who passed away during the writing of this book. He was a teacher at heart and taught me about the joy that helping others can bring. He also always told me that I could achieve anything I set my mind to, and I always believed him.

A special thank you to all the families of children with autism spectrum disorder who have allowed me to be a part of their life. I have learned so much from you, and these experiences are why I feel so passionately about working with children with autism spectrum disorder. Every day you inspire me to continue to learn more and be a partner in your successes. In particular, I extend gratitude to the families of the children in the various case studies in this book who have generously shared their experiences with us.

I would also like to express appreciation to all of my colleagues at the University of South Florida. I enjoy our collaborations, and they have helped me develop my knowledge and clinical skills. Thanks to Sylvia Diehl for fostering my passion in working with the families of children with autism spectrum disorder, Elaine Silliman for always sharing her vast knowledge, and Ruth Bahr for being the first to fan the flames of my interest in research.

Finally, this book could not have been created without the support of my entire family. My wonderful husband, R. P., offered unending support, including giving me the gift of time to pursue this endeavor. He took care of our girls while I wrote during many nights and weekends. I am lucky to have a husband who makes my happiness and success a priority. My daughter, Julia, waited patiently many times while being told "mommy is writing her book." My mother, Joanne, and sister, Vanessa, selflessly donated many hours of their time to help watch the girls, so that I could steal some uninterrupted writing time. The contributions of all of my family, including mother-in-law, Patti, and stepfather, Tom, were instrumental in the completion of this project. Thank you and I love you all.

—Michelle Peters Hite, MS, CCC-SLP

CHAPTER

1

An Overview of Autism Spectrum Disorder

Introduction

Snapshots of Individuals with Autism Spectrum Disorder

Case A: FG-Male, 6 Years Old, Diagnosis: Autism

Finnegan's Story, written by his dad, Sean

Finnegan can talk. When I arrive at home after work, he says, "Hi, Daddy." When I ask him if he's hungry, he says, "Grilled cheese." For me and my wife, this is nothing short of amazing. To an outsider, hearing Finn utter these words might seem common place—an everyday greeting, a simple yet appropriate answer to a question. However, for us, his ability to effectively communicate his thoughts marks a milestone in his life.

Finnegan is now six years old, but it wasn't very long ago that the question, "Are you hungry" would be answered by spinning the tires of a toy car or staring at the ceiling fan. The crickets were chirping for years. It is probably obvious that Finnegan's journey to realize his voice was not an easy one. As an infant and toddler, he missed almost all of the normal developmental benchmarks. He crawled and walked late. He didn't seek out eye contact. His play was rarely, if ever, imaginative.

A funny thing happens to the people around you when your child begins missing mile-stones. "Oh, he hasn't begun to talk yet?" one might ask. "That's perfectly normal. Your cousin didn't talk until . . . " Although these types of questions and responses are well-intentioned, meant to make one feel that everything is on track, the problem is that the avoidance of addressing what is really going on is pervasive. When discussing concerns

1

about Finnegan, we received these types of responses across the board—from our family, friends and, worse, from multiple pediatricians. Because I was hearing reports from our support network and even from doctors that everything was fine, I crept into a state of denial, blocking out what I knew to be true—that our son's development was delayed. Finn's mother, thankfully, persevered and sought out answers as to why Finn was so developmentally behind other children his age.

Search after search on the Internet all pointed my wife to the same word: autism. And, after finding experts in the diagnostic tools to recognize autism, we were finally presented with an official diagnosis. What did that mean for Finn's future? We are still figuring out the answers to that question. However, the immediate reaction to such a diagnosis was to try to fix things—to try to help Finnegan attain the tools he needs to have the best life possible.

Finnegan carried many of the traits associated with autism in young children. In addition to being behind his peers developmentally, Finnegan also exhibited frequent tantrums or *meltdowns*, had issues with fine and gross motor control, and, as we would later learn, had apraxia, a secondary but related condition affecting his speech abilities. All of these traits lent difficulty to our approaches to help Finnegan. For example, how were we going to attempt to help Finnegan focus on our efforts to teach him to talk when: (1) he is prone to meltdown if any of his surroundings change; (2) he will not make eye contact or focus on any task that doesn't involve spinning tires; and (3) his mouth doesn't seem to work properly enough to form words? The list could go on. We needed help, and that help came in the form of speech language pathologists, applied behavior analysis (ABA) therapists, and resources from the Center for Autism and Related Disorders (CARD) and other avenues.

Finnegan's mother and I learned very quickly about the different schools of thought associated with autism therapy. Were we going to implement the Floortime/DIR model or move toward applied behavior analysis? Ultimately, we decided that it was in Finnegan's best interests to keep an open mind and coordinate an interdisciplinary approach to his therapy that utilized many different techniques but targeted the specific problems Finnegan was experiencing. Soon after his diagnosis, the walls of our home were filled with data charts, Picture Exchange Communication Systems (PECS), notes from therapists, and stacks upon stacks of books about autism.

Our family spent years with various therapists and students working with Finnegan in our home and in clinical settings. With their help, Finnegan graduated from PECS to typing and spelling words, using augmentative speech devices and, finally, to verbalizing simple requests. The most effective clinicians and students in helping Finnegan through this journey were those who took the time to not only get to know all they could about Finnegan and the issues with which he was struggling, but also learn how much his parents knew about the therapeutic methodologies they were utilizing, what level of involvement the parents had in therapy when clinicians were not present, what other therapists working with Finnegan were doing, and so forth. In other words, the best therapists were those who took a type of holistic approach to get the big picture of what was going on with Finnegan and his family. These therapists learned up front about the parents' knowledge of autism and therapeutic interventions, so there was no session time wasted in reiterating to the parents what was at stake in, say, the redirection of problematic behaviors.

Finnegan can talk. He is an incredibly smart and loving kid and has come miles. However, his journey is not yet complete. He will likely encounter many more therapists on his path to discover a stronger voice and to navigate the complex world of human social interaction. For Finnegan to succeed, he will need a strong network of effective clinicians who work with each other and our family to root out a kind of holistic therapeutic approach that takes into account much more than the successes and failures that take place in a single therapy session.

Case B: AH-Female, 9 Years Old, Diagnosis: Autism

Avery's Story, taken from an interview with Avery's mom, Shena

Q: How did you know to seek a diagnosis?

A: When I searched the Internet for Avery's amazing gifts as an 18-month-old, one thing that came up was hyperlexia. This is an unusual genius understanding of letters and numbers—it is also a splinter skill of autism. This led me to look out for signs of autism. She was just under age 2 when the autism regression started.

Q: What was that like as a parent going through the diagnostic process and aftermath?

A: The first thing I had to learn was if it was even the right choice to go after a diagnosis. I mean, no one wants their child to be labeled, right? I learned quickly that the label was the key to services, help, and understanding. It was the best thing I could do for her.

The next thing I learned was that early intervention was very important, so that time in our lives turned into a time-sucking flurry of research, therapy, and advocacy.

The difficult part was the strong, conflicting opinions about autism I came across in my research, like the raging vaccination debate and the gluten-free diet. I learned, after eight years, that there is a truth to both sides. I also learned that I knew what was best for my child—to learn from my mistakes, to advocate beyond what was comfortable for anyone, and most of all, to trust my gut. What a crash course in motherhood!

Q: What was the most helpful and challenging part of the entire process?

A: The most helpful part of the process was that my husband, Jeff, was on board and supportive of all of my research. The other helpful part was CARD (Center for Autism and Related Disabilities). When we moved to Gainesville, we contacted them, and it was like we found a family there to guide us through this whole autism business. At CARD, there were real people at a real location who you could speak to and learn from. It was such a relief to have them there. CARD helped navigate the developmental skills. Jeff and I attended parent/child communication classes and potty training classes. One of the CARD consultants, Cathy Zenko, came and spoke to Avery's first grade class about what autism was, and in 15 minutes, changed how her classmates perceived her and how they treated her for the rest of the year. Cathy came back and did it again the next year too.

Q: How is Avery doing now?

A: Now, Avery is in fourth grade with her peers. Her classmates and teachers understand her, so when she has a hard time focusing or processing what is being asked of her, she doesn't get in trouble. She is a very intelligent, perceptive, and kind little girl. She has friends in her class who care about her, and no one makes fun of her challenges. She is known in her class for her amazing fiction stories that she reads out to the class when they are asked to share. She also is known for her wonderful drawings and comic strips.

Her biggest challenge is taking her folder out of her backpack, hanging up her backpack, putting away her lunchbox, and getting a chair and sitting at her desk in the morning. She can do multiplication and early algebra problems just fine.

Q: How did Avery's diagnosis impact the family?

A: Avery and autism fit right in with our family just fine. She is the oldest of three, and her siblings are "typical"—whatever that means. The kids get along well; they play and they fight. I suppose the unusual part is how we don't eat out often as we have found the gluten-free, casein-free, and even soy-free diet, helps Avery focus. We eat organic food with no preservatives; we try and stay away from anything processed, and we don't eat fast food.

Q: What are your goals and dreams for Avery?

A: She now has things that I have always wanted for her. She has friends, a great education, a great school, cute clothes, extracurricular activities, and a family who loves and supports her. In my opinion, she is a very fortunate little girl—autism or no autism. If I may ask for more, I would like for her to have better eye contact and to not slip away into her own world so often . . .

I hope Avery finds love and a husband and maybe even has children someday. I hope she goes on to college and someday finds a job she enjoys where she can contribute her intelligence (I'm thinking medical research or art.) Whatever she chooses, I am sure she will be amazing at it. She is beautiful, kind, and brilliant. She has the world at her fingertips; she has her family, and she has CARD.

Q: What does a speech therapist need to know about Avery to help provide meaningful intervention?

A: She learns best one-on-one. She learns better one-on-one, than in social skills groups where her peers have autism spectrum disorder. She learns best doing role playing with dolls. Avery is more empathetic than most kids on the spectrum. Don't push her too far. If she isn't listening, she is having a bad sensory day. It is not because she is misbehaving. Finally, she is very smart;

the ADD portion of her disability is the most distracting for her at this point, and she has trouble focusing on tasks that she doesn't feel confident. I'd also like to tell you three things that are important to me personally . . .

1. *Diet*
2. *Reversability?*
3. *Autism . . . not autistic*

1. *Changing Avery's diet has helped her a lot. This is met with skepticism by many, but her whole personality can be changed, for example, by sugar. (When her siblings have sugar, it doesn't seem to affect them at all.) I think this food issue is being touched upon lightly (GFCF) but is much bigger and more important than is being reported, or perhaps discovered at this time. Perhaps in the future that will change.*

2. *Avery's doctor says she "hints at reversibility" mostly because she sheds her symptoms when she has a fever and because Methyl-B12 shots do wonders for her. Although we enjoy having hope that there will be a cure for her barriers someday, we are not crippled by that hope. We are inspired that there is a perhaps out there, while being wildly proud of who she is . . . with autism.*

3. *Has autism not autistic. (It may sound like nitpicking but it's not . . . and here is why.)*

I prefer that Avery is described as "having autism," rather than "autistic." This is an important distinction to me because I don't think that autism should define a person completely. Yes, it is best to have a diagnosis, as this helps the public understand better how to empathize and treat a person with autism. But for example, when a person has cancer, we don't call them, canceric. We call them a cancer patient or say they have cancer, because cancer is not who they are.

To sum it up, saying a person has autism sounds to me like they are an individual who happens to be dealing with the barriers that autism presents. But describing a person as Autistic, conjures up an often inaccurate picture of what we may imagine autism to be (Rainman to start with) and leaves out the fact that kids and adults on the autism spectrum are widely varied individuals with their own personalities.

Based on the two cases presented above, it is apparent that the face of autism spectrum disorder (ASD) can present quite differently. Similarly, wide disparity can be observed in each family's journey to diagnosis. The autism spectrum involves a broad range of characteristics, however, core features do exist within the profiles of all individuals diagnosed with ASD.

Autism Spectrum Disorder (ASD)

Do I Really Need to Know About ASD?

Based on the current prevalence statistics stating that 1 out of 88 children have a diagnosis of ASD (Centers for Disease Control and Prevention, 2012), any speech-language pathologist (SLP) working with the pediatric population needs to know what ASD is. The results from the American Speech-Language-Hearing Association (2011) SLP Health Care Survey Report state, that "overall, children with autism accounted for 20% of SLPs' caseloads in 2011, up considerably from 6% in 2009. Percentages were highest in pediatric hospitals, home health, and outpatient clinics and offices" (p. 3). Therefore, it is important for SLPs to be knowledgeable of the characteristics associated with ASDs.

SLPs are often part of a multidisciplinary diagnostic team as the communication and social interaction expert. Because communication delays are usually the first sign parents recognize, the SLP is often the first person the parents confront with the question, "Do you think my child has autism?" or "Why isn't my child talking?" In order to answer these questions, the SLP needs to have a firm understanding of the diagnostic characteristics of ASD to provide the parents with an honest, evidence-based response to their concerns. Therefore, it is paramount that SLPs, especially those serving the pediatric population, are familiar with the most current diagnostic tools and checklists used to identify ASD. The *Diagnostic Statistical Manual* (DSM-IV-TR; American Psychiatric Association, 2000) or the recently updated fifth edition (DSM-5), released in May 2013, are important references to have. For children ages 24 to 36 months, the *Systematic Observation of Red Flags for Young Children* (SORF; McCoy, Wetherby, & Woods, 2009; Wetherby, Woods, Allen, Cleary, Dickinson, & Lord, 2004) is a parent-friendly checklist that can serve as the SLP's guide in discussing concerns parents bring up as they relate to signs or symptoms of ASD.

ASD: What Is It?

ASD is a neurodevelopmental disorder characterized by significant difficulties in the areas of social interaction, communication, and restricted and repetitive interests, behaviors, and/or activities, according to the *Diagnostic and Statistical Manual of Mental Disorders—IV* (DSM-IV-TR; American Psychiatric Association, 2000). The National Research Council (2001) noted, "Autism spectrum disorders are present from birth or very early in development and affect essential human behaviors such as social interaction, the ability to communicate ideas and feelings, imagination, and the establishment of relationships with others" (p. 1). Some of the earliest signs of ASD seen between the first and second years of life are lack of joint attention and failure to respond to name when called (McCoy et al., 2009; Osterling & Dawson, 1994; Wetherby et al., 2004). These signs coupled with a delay in verbal language often drive parents to seek answers that lead to a diagnosis of ASD.

The DSM-IV-TR provides the diagnostic criteria that has been used since 2000 by physicians to diagnose individuals with ASD. However, it is important to note the *Diagnostic and Statistical Manual of Mental Disorders—5* (DSM-5) was released in May, 2013. The criteria found in both the DSM-IV-TR and the DSM-5 are reviewed and compared in the following section.

DSM-IV-TR Guidelines

The DSM-IV-TR guidelines set forth by the American Psychiatric Association (2000) describe autism spectrum disorders as referring to a group of related pervasive developmental disorders (PDD) that share underlying core difficulties within the following three domains: (1) social interaction, (2) communication, and (3) restricted, repetitive, and stereotyped patterns of behaviors, interests, and activities (Figure 1–1). This group includes the following diagnostic categories: autistic disorder, Asperger disorder, pervasive developmental disorders not otherwise specified (PDD-NOS), Rett's disorder, and childhood disintegrative disorder. Each category has a specific formula of diagnostic criteria (Table 1–1). For example, for a diagnosis of autistic disorder, six or more items listed in the areas of social interaction, communication, and restricted and repetitive behaviors or interests must be present, specifically, at least two criteria from the social domain and at least one in the communication and behavior domains (American Psychiatric Association, 2000, p. 75).

DSM-5 Guidelines

The DSM-5 defines autism spectrum disorder as one unified spectrum with a range of difficulty associated with two core features instead of the previous model of three core areas of impairment (American Psychiatric Association, 2013). The DSM-5 combines the domains of impairments in social interaction and communication into the same general category and keeps the restricted, repetitive, and stereotyped patterns of behaviors, interests, and activities domain (Figure 1–2). Although ASD now stands as one unifying construct, it is still acknowledged that an incredible range exists within the autism spectrum (American Psychiatric Association, 2013).

Although the clinical diagnosis is moving to one unified classification, the DSM-5 does incorporate ways to represent the range of symptoms expressed by assigning severity levels and other clinical specifiers (American Psychiatric Association, 2013; Wetherby, 2012). Rather than provide separate clinical diagnoses to represent variations of ASD, the evaluators are to describe how each domain is affected uniquely in individuals with ASD (Wetherby, 2012). Descriptions of *severity level* are made based on the child's support level needs. It is important to note that the severity levels are described based on the level of functional presentation and support needs within the community rather than formal testing levels—for example, IQ test results, formal language score results, and so forth (American Psychiatric Association, 2013; Wetherby, 2012). Three severity levels are described, including Levels 1, 2, and 3. These levels are assigned to each of the two component areas (social/communication and restricted/repetitive behavior) individually and describe functional support needs in each area. Level 3 refers to individuals "requiring very substantial support," including individuals with little initiation or response for social communication or extreme difficulty redirecting from rituals, preoccupation, or repetitive behaviors. Level 2 refers to individuals "requiring substantial support" due to difficulties with social communication despite supports being in place. Less difficulty is noted with redirection from rituals, preoccupations, or repetitive behaviors, but the individual continues to present with significant difficulty in this area. Finally, Level 1 describes those individuals who "require support" with: (1) initiating social communication to typical levels, despite support and (2) disruption of daily functioning due to presence of rituals and repetitive behaviors and interests.

Table 1–1. DSM-IV-TR Guidelines (American Psychiatric Association, 2000)

	Pervasive Developmental Disorders (PDD)			
	Autism Spectrum Disorders			
Autistic Disorder	Asperger's Disorder	Pervasive Developmental Disorder—Not Otherwise Specified (PDD-NOS)	Rett's Disorder	Childhood Disintegrative Disorder (CDD)

Impairments in Three Domains:

(#1) Social Interaction	(#2) Communication	(#3) Restricted, Repetitive, and Stereotyped Patterns of Behaviors, Interests, and Activities
• Marked impairment in the use of multiple nonverbal behaviors such as eye-to-eye gaze, facial expression, body postures, and gestures to regulate social interaction • Failure to develop peer relationships appropriate to developmental level • Lack of spontaneous seeking to share enjoyment, interests, or achievements with other people • Lack of social or emotional reciprocity	• Delay in, or total lack of, development of spoken language (not accompanied by an attempt to compensate through alternative modes of communication such as gesture or mime) • Marked impairment in initiating or sustaining a conversation (adequate speech) • Stereotyped and repetitive use of language or idiosyncratic language • Lack of varied, spontaneous make-believe play or social imitative play appropriate to developmental level	• Encompassing preoccupation with one or more stereotyped and restricted patterns of interest; abnormal intensity or focus • Inflexible adherence to specific, nonfunctional routines or rituals • Stereotyped and repetitive motor mannerisms • Persistent preoccupation with parts of objects

Autistic Disorder:	Asperger's Disorder:	PDD-NOS:	Rett's Disorder:	CDD:
• Total of 6 or more items	• ≥2 from #1	• Criteria not met for a specific PDD	A. All following normal:	• Normal development at least 2 years after birth
• ≥2 items from 1	• At least 1 from #3	• Used when a severe and pervasive impairment exists in #1; also #2 or #3	• Prenatal and perinatal development	• Significant loss of previously acquired skills before age 10 years in ≥2 of these: Expressive or receptive language, social skills or adaptive behavior, bowel or bladder control, play, and motor skills
• ≥1 item from 2	• Impairment seen in social, occupational, or other important areas of functioning	• Category also includes atypical autism; may be late age of onset for autistic disorder, atypical symptomatology, or subthreshold symptomatology	• Psychomotor development <5 months of age	• ≥2 from the above areas #1, #2, or #3
• ≥1 item from 3	• No clinically significant general delay in language		• Head circumference at birth	
• Delays in one of the following prior to age 3 years: social interaction, language as used in social communication, or symbolic or imaginative play	• No clinically significant delay in cognitive development, self-help skills, adaptive behavior		B. After period of normal development:	
			• Deceleration of head growth (5–48 months)	
			• Loss of previously acquired purposeful hand skills (5–30 months); development of stereotyped hand movements	
			• Loss of social engagement	
			• Poorly coordinated gait or trunk movements	
			• Severely impaired expressive and receptive language development with severe psychomotor retardation	

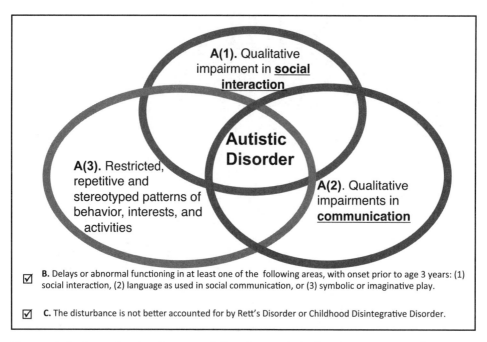

Figure 1–1. Pervasive developmental disorder: Autistic disorder DSM-IV-TR (American Psychiatric Association, 2000). This figure illustrates the diagnostic criteria for autistic disorder according to the DSM-IV-TR.

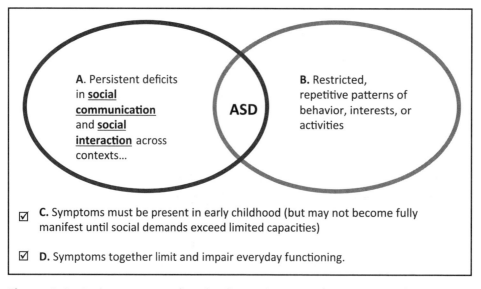

Figure 1–2. Autism spectrum disorder diagnosis: DSM-5 (American Psychiatric Association, 2013). This figure illustrates the diagnostic criteria for autism spectrum disorder under the new DSM-5 guidelines.

Professionals who have experience working with individuals with ASD are intensely aware of the variability in profiles. For instance, in the social communication realm, some individuals with ASD can present with very little verbal communication, whereas others can present with excessive verbal communication but have difficulty in the areas of understanding social, conversational rules for using language in everyday social communication. Although the DSM-5 (2013) criteria specify that the symptoms of ASD must be present in early childhood, it is noted that at times the symptoms may not be detected until later until "social demands exceed limited capacities." This might be particularly important to remember when encountering children presenting with *milder* forms of ASD, including those previously diagnosed with Asperger Disorder. Care must be taken to ensure that young children and individuals with less obvious forms of ASD are not denied support because their needs may not be as evident to the untrained observer.

Table 1–2 outlines the DSM-5 guidelines that all children diagnosed with ASD must now demonstrate to receive a diagnosis.

Table 1–2. Criteria for ASD According to DSM-5 (2013)

Pervasive Developmental Disorders					
Autism Spectrum Disorder					
Impairments in Two Domains:					

A) Social communication:			B) Restricted, repetitive patterns of behavior, interests, or activities (at least two of the following):		
✓ Deficits in social-emotional reciprocity ✓ Deficits in nonverbal communicative behaviors used for social interaction ✓ Deficits in developing and maintaining relationships, appropriate to developmental level and beyond those with caregivers			✓ Stereotyped or repetitive speech, motor movements, or use of objects ✓ Inflexible adherence to routines, ritualized patterns of verbal or nonverbal behavior, or insistence on sameness ✓ Highly restricted, fixated interests that are abnormal in intensity or focus ✓ Hyper-or hyporeactivity to sensory input or unusual interest in sensory aspects of environment		
Severity Level for (A):			**Severity Level for (B):**		
Level 1	Level 2	Level 3	Level 1	Level 2	Level 3
Requiring support	Requiring substantial support	Requiring very substantial support	Requiring support	Requiring substantial support	Requiring very substantial support

The following conditions also must be met:

C) Present in early childhood, but may not have fully manifested until social demands exceeded limited capacities

D) Limits and impairs everyday functioning (social, occupational)

Summary of Significant Proposed DSM-5 Changes:

- Combination of the social and communication domains into one. Overall, the DSM-5 contains two domains instead of three domains. The DSM-IV-TR refers to a three-domain model, whereas the DSM-5 describes a two-domain model (see Figures 1–1 and 1–2 for comparison).

- Condensing autistic disorder, Asperger disorder, PDD-NOS, and childhood disintegrative disorder into one inclusive diagnosis of autism spectrum disorder. These previous subtypes are grouped together as one, singular autism spectrum disorder.

- Reorganization and further development of symptoms within the domains. An important highlight is that the restricted, repetitive behavior domain now includes a description of possible sensory processing differences.

- A severity level is individually given to the two main components of ASD, which is based on functional support needs.

Additional Changes Within the DSM-5: Communication Disorders

Important changes are also noted within the diagnostic category of Communication Disorders. Several disorders are included underneath the category of Communication Disorder, including Social (Pragmatic) Language Disorder. Social (pragmatic) language disorder is present when difficulties are experienced in the "social use of verbal and nonverbal communication" which lead to functional deficits in "social participation, social relationships, academic achievement, or occupational performance" (American Psychiatric Association, 2013, pp. 47–48). Clinicians may see individuals who previously fell under the category of PDD-NOS being diagnosed with social (pragmatic) communication disorder (Wetherby, 2012) if the child only displays the social communication delays without the presence of the restricted, repetitive, and stereotypic behaviors and interests. The DSM-5 (2013) notes within the criteria for social (pragmatic) communication disorder that the symptoms noted by the clinician should not be better explained by autism spectrum disorder. It is imperative that the professionals carefully evaluate if a child may have a milder form of ASD that is presenting like a social (pragmatic) communication disorder in order to ensure that child receives the right supports and services.

Summary: The ASD Diagnosis and the SLP

The SLP should be aware of the different aspects and rationales for giving diagnoses according to both DSM-IV-TR and DSM-5 guidelines. Even though the DSM-5 guidelines have been released, SLPs will still see children referred for therapy based on an ASD diagnosis that was determined under the DSM-IV-TR guidelines. Knowledge of the basis for diagnosis of an autism spectrum disorder, including the diagnostic categories from the DSM-IV-TR of Asperger disorder, PDD-NOS, and childhood disintegrative disorder, will enable the SLP to understand the individual's presenting profile at the time of evaluation and diagnosis. It is important to note that despite the route and method of diagnosis, the core symptoms related to a diagnosis of ASD remain. Regardless of the incoming diagnosis, it is always important to remember to use person-first language when referring to any individual. In other words, always list the individual first, followed by the diagnosis. For example, instead of saying "an autistic person," "an autistic," and so forth, refer to individuals as a "person with autism/ASD."

Cognitive Characteristics and Learning Styles of Individuals with ASD

The SLP who plans to provide quality intervention to individuals on the autism spectrum needs to understand the basic diagnostic criteria and how they affect the way individuals with ASD think, learn, and communicate. Individuals with ASD present a unique set of cognitive characteristics that are important for the SLP to understand, so they can provide intervention that targets the underpinnings of the language, learning, and social communication impairments. The differences in the development of theory of mind (or perspective taking), executive function, central coherence, emotion regulation, and play are important characteristics for the SLP to consider when developing a therapy plan targeting observed deficits in oral, written and social communication. These difficulties often have significant impacts on learning in a group educational setting as well. Although difficulties in these areas may not be part of the core features used to diagnose ASD, they are frequently observed and often play a significant role in the individual's overall success in daily life. This includes success within the home and community environments, as well as learning outcomes in academic settings.

Theory of Mind or Perspective Taking

This is often described as a key feature explaining the underlying reason for social communication deficits observed. Theory of mind is the ability to understand others' thoughts, feelings, beliefs, and desires (Baron-Cohen, 1989, 2000; Baron-Cohen, Leslie, & Frith, 1985; Frith, 1989). The ability to take the perspectives of others, read their emotions, and change your behavior to match the emotions of others is a documented area of weakness in people with ASD (Baron-Cohen, 1989; Baron-Cohen et al., 1985; Frith, 1989; Myles & Southwick, 1999).

Difficulty in perspective taking affects students with ASD's ability to understand "the hidden curriculum" (Myles, Schelvan, & Trautman, 2004). Myles et al. (2004) describe the hidden curriculum as those social rules people just know, but are never taught. They are invisible; however, obeying these hidden rules is, in part, what makes a person socially successful. The literal nature of students with ASD, along with their need to process things visually and their extreme difficulty understanding and reading others' emotions, is a recipe for social disaster (Zenko, 2011). Therefore, understanding the underlying social pragmatic weaknesses common in individuals with ASD is imperative to creating and implementing a successful treatment plan. See Chapters 3 and 5 for more information on assessment and treatment of social communication difficulties.

Executive Function

Executive function (EF) refers to an individual's ability to utilize higher-order cognitive skills to integrate and coordinate basic cognitive functions such as perception, attention, and memory (Baron, 2004). Denckla (1989) defines EF as the ability to plan and sequence behaviors, attend to multiple sources of information simultaneously, understand the overall meaning of situations, resist distractions, suppress inappropriate responses, and remain on task for prolonged periods of time. Baron's (2004) definition is similar; "EF emphasizes the metacognitive capacities that allow an individual to perceive stimuli from his or her environment, respond adaptively, flexibly change direction, anticipate future goals, consider consequences, and respond in an integrated or common-sense way, utilizing all these capacities to serve a common purposive goal" (p. 135).

Individuals with ASD have difficulty with almost all components of the above definitions, thus creating challenges in multiple areas (Joseph & Tager-Flusberg, 2004; McEvoy, Rogers, & Pennington, 1993; Ozonoff & McEvoy, 1994; Ozonoff, Pennington, & Rogers, 1991). As an SLP, the areas of executive function that are most likely to be a focus of any language session include, but are not limited to: shifting attention, determining what is the most important stimuli to pay attention to in any situation, understanding the gist or main idea of complex situations, learning what is appropriate to say and do, controlling impulses, and making logical and socially acceptable decisions. Executive function is something most individuals take for granted and learn incidentally. This is one more example of hidden skills that are not learned automatically for individuals with ASD and have a significant impact on their success. Therefore, SLPs need to understand the importance of EF and help individuals with ASD learn how to improve this complex metacognitive process (Joseph & Tager-Flusberg, 2004; McEvoy et al., 1993; Ozonoff & McEvoy, 1994; Ozonoff et al., 1991).

Central Coherence

Individuals with ASD often have difficulty with central coherence, which is an impairment in general information processing or gestalt thinking (Frith, 1989; Happé, 1997). In other words, they have difficulty determining the big picture and tend to focus on discrete and highly specific details. This difficulty in understanding the main idea or overall gist has significant repercussions on learning new concepts, conversational skills, and reading comprehension.

One analogy to explain central coherence is the zoom feature seen on cameras and web-based maps. Weak central coherence is like having the camera zoomed in all the time, highlighting the tiny details, but not being able to recognize what the picture is. Noticing details is important, but it must be paired with the ability to *zoom out* and see how the small details contribute to the larger, complete concept. Figure 1–3 illustrates what

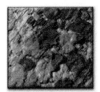

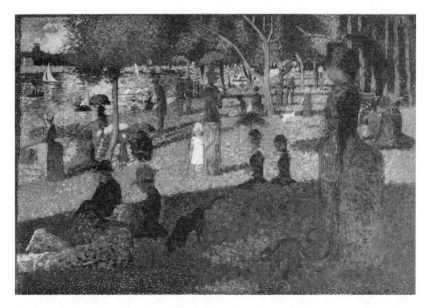

Figure 1–3. Illustration of central coherence using the classic painting, Sunday Afternoon on the Island Grand Jatte, by George Seurat. This figure illustrates the concept of weak central coherence. The work of art depicted in this image and the reproduction thereof are in the public domain worldwide. The reproduction is part of a collection of reproductions compiled by The Yorck Project. The compilation copyright is held by Zenodot Verlagsgesellschaft mbH and licensed under the GNU Free Documentation License.

happens if you zoom in too close (the picture on the left); the meaning of the painting is lost because the view is on the very specific components, or dots, in the picture. This is a parallel to weak central coherence. In contrast, when the picture is viewed farther away, the overall meaning and purpose of the dots can be seen (right); strong central coherence. The ability to summarize, extract the main idea, and make connections regarding how things go together requires a strong central coherence. As an SLP, focusing on directly teaching association, summarization, and main idea concepts is necessary for individuals with ASD to improve both oral and written communication.

Emotional Regulation

All individuals have varying abilities to control their own internal emotional state (Prizant, Wetherby, Rubin, Laurent, & Rydell, 2006). Children with ASD often have significant difficulty regulating and communicating their own internal emotional states and being available for learning. Although these emotional regulation or sensory processing difficulties were viewed as secondary to the core characteristics of ASD, the impact of difficulties with emotional regulation can significantly affect daily functioning and learning (Prizant et al., 2006). It is important to note that the new definition of ASD found in the DSM-5 (2013) includes sensory processing differences within the diagnostic characteristics of "Restricted, repetitive patterns of behavior, interests, or activities."

Emotional regulation difficulties may be secondary to one or more of a variety of underlying factors, including: frustration with understanding social conventions and interpersonal experiences; communication challenges; reactions to sensory processing differences, sleep, and feeding problems; and motor planning difficulties leading to trouble with speech and executing gross motor movements (Prizant & Meyer, 1993; Prizant et al., 2006). Increased rates of coexisting anxiety and depression in this population can also affect their ability to maintain internal homeostasis (Attwood, 2004; Kim, Szatmari, Bryson, Streiner, & Wilson, 2000; Klin, Pauls, Schultz, & Volkmar, 2005). Recognizing the signs and symptoms of anxiety and depression is crucial for SLPs, so they can refer individuals to the proper medical provider(s) to monitor the coexisting mental health concerns.

Klinger and Dawson (1992) summarized research findings on the reception and processing problems seen in autism, finding that children with autism fail to orient, process, and respond to new and unpredictable stimuli or events in the same way as their typically developing peers. This "abnormal orienting response may be related to difficulties in arousal regulation" (Klinger & Dawson, 1992, p. 164). They hypothesize that "children with autism have an unusually narrow range of optimal stimulation" (Klinger & Dawson, 1992, p. 165), ranging between a lower level that doesn't register with the child at all; to a narrow, slightly higher level that enables the child to orient, attend, and respond adaptively; to an upper level that causes overarousal, confusion, and aversion or avoidance. Prizant et al. (2006) noted that children with emotional states at either extreme are "often at the mercy of overwhelming reactions such as anxiety, fear, distress, or even dysregulating positive emotional states of elation and giddiness" (p. 5).

The negative impact of the sensory processing challenges along with the narrow window of optimal attention is critical for providers to understand when working with individuals on the autism spectrum. Stress from the constant feeling of overarousal or difficulty with raising arousal level enough to actively engage can make learning nearly impossible and exhausting. Therefore, making sure to acknowledge and address individuals' arousal levels and sensory overload is the first step any therapist should take before expecting any meaningful learning to occur.

Play Development

Play development is an important skill related to the development of both the symbolic and the social aspects of language development (Prizant et al., 2006). Children with ASD exhibit difficulties with play development due to a culmination of the core features and cognitive characteristics previously discussed. According to the DSM-IV-TR, children with ASD might demonstrate "lack of varied, spontaneous make-believe play or social imitative play appropriate to developmental level" (American Psychiatric Association, 2000, p. 75).

Play development and social communication are inextricably tied (Westby, 1988). The development of more elaborate and complex play experiences offers rich opportunities for the development of social communication in naturalistic situations. For example, playing restaurant develops both symbolic play skills as well as language routines commonly used within a familiar setting. This is even more important when working with children with ASD due to inherent difficulty generalizing information (National Research

Council, 2001). Due to the fundamental connections of play and language development, the SLP plays an important role in assessing the components of play of children with ASD and helping design individualized treatment plans that address the underlying aspects of difficulty with play development (see Chapters 3 and 5 for more information about assessment and intervention of play).

Summary: How Does the SLP Fit into the ASD Puzzle?

SLPs play an integral role in working with children on the autism spectrum. With the social communication impairment being one of the first noticeable signs of ASD, the SLP is often one of the first professionals parents seek when they have concerns regarding their child's development. Ideally, SLPs are included on any multidisciplinary diagnostic team so he or she can provide valuable information about the social and communication development of the person being evaluated. Understanding the diagnostic characteristics associated with ASD is important for any SLP who plans to work with the pediatric population because the prevalence rate for this particular disorder is now 1 out of 88 children (Centers for Disease Control and Prevention, 2012). In keeping with the general increase in prevalence, SLPs have seen increased numbers of children with ASD on their caseloads (Hasselkus, 2011). According to a recent American Speech-Language-Hearing Association health care survey, SLPs reported that children with ASD made up 20% of their caseloads, as compared with the 6% that was reported back in 2009 (American Speech-Language-Hearing Association, 2011). This vast spectrum of individuals has a unique set of strengths and challenges which, once understood, can thrive with skilled intervention. Therefore, it is imperative that any SLP working with children on the spectrum carefully assess and understand how ASD affects each child so that the underlying deficits can be targeted in an autism-friendly manner to achieve successful outcomes.

Learning Tool

1. Name the core features associated with a diagnosis of ASD.

2. Name and describe two other cognitive characteristics associated with ASD. How might these characteristics relate to the development of language?

3. Explain the relationship between the development of play and communication. Why is it important to target play skills within intervention for social communication?

Useful Websites

- American Psychiatric Association DSM-5 website: http://www.dsm5.org

- American Speech-Language-Hearing Association Practice Policies:
  - Principles for Speech-Language Pathologists in Diagnosis, Assessment, and Treatment of Autism Spectrum Disorders across the Life Span: http://www.asha.org/docs/html/TR2006-00143.html
  - Guidelines for Speech-Language Pathologists in Diagnosis, Assessment, and Treatment of Autism Spectrum Disorders across the Life Span: http://www.asha.org/docs/html/GL2006-00049.html
- Autism Navigator: http://med.fsu.edu/index.cfm?page=autismInstitute.autismNavigator
- Autism Speaks: http://www.autismspeaks.org/
- Autism Society of America: http://www.autism-society.org/
- Centers for Disease Control and Prevention, information regarding autism spectrum disorders: http://www.cdc.gov/ncbddd/autism/index.html
- First Signs, Video Glossary: https://www.firstsigns.org/asd_video_glossary/asdvg_about.htm
- First Words Project: http://firstwords.fsu.edu/
- National Institute of Mental Health: http://www.nimh.nih.gov/health/publications/autism-listing.shtml
- The Florida Centers for Autism and Related Disabilities: http://florida-card.org/

References

American Psychiatric Association. (2000). *Diagnostic and statistical manual of mental disorders* (4th ed., Text rev.). Washington, DC: Author.

American Psychiatric Association. (2013). *Diagnostic and statistical manual of mental health disorders: DSM-5* (5th ed.). Washington, DC: American Psychiatric Publishing.

American Speech-Language-Hearing Association. (2011). *SLP health care survey report: Patient caseload characteristics trends, 2005–2011*. Retrieved from http://www.asha.org

Attwood, T. (2004). Cognitive behaviour therapy for children and adults with Asperger's syndrome. *Behaviour Change, 21*(3), 147–161.

Baron, I. S. (2004). *Neuropsychological evaluation of the child*. Oxford, UK: Oxford University Press.

Baron-Cohen, S. (1989). The autistic child's theory of mind: A case of specific developmental delay. *Journal of Child Psychology and Psychiatry, 30*(2), 285–297.

Baron-Cohen, S. (2000). Theory of mind and autism: A fifteen year review. In S. Baron-Cohen, H. Tager-Flusberg, & D. J. Cohen (Eds.), *Understanding other minds: Perspectives from developmental cognitive neuroscience* (pp. 3–20). Oxford, UK: Oxford University Press.

Baron-Cohen, S., Leslie, A. M., & Frith, U. (1985). Does the autistic child have a "theory of mind"? *Cognition, 21*, 37–46.

Centers for Disease Control and Prevention. (2012). Prevalence of autism spectrum disorders—Autism and developmental disabilities monitoring network, United States, 2008. *Morbidity and Mortal Weekly Report (MMWR), 61*(SS03). Retrieved from http://www.cdc.gov/ncbddd/autism/documents/ADDM-2012-Community-Report.pdf

Denckla, M. B. (1989). Executive function, the overlap zone between attention deficit hyperactivity disorder and learning disabilities. *International Pediatrics, 4*, 155–160.

Frith, U. (1989). Autism and "theory of mind." In C. Gillberg (Ed.), *Diagnosis and treatment of autism* (pp. 33–52). New York, NY: Plenum Press.

Happé, F. G. E. (1997). Central coherence and theory of mind in autism: Reading homographs in context. *British Journal of Developmental Psychology, 15*(1), 1–12.

Hasselkus, A. (2011, October 11). What's happening in health care: 2011 survey results. *ASHA Leader.*

Joseph, R. M., & Tager-Flusberg, H. (2004). The relationship of theory of mind and executive functions to symptom type and severity in children with autism. *Developmental Psychopathology, 16*(1), 137–155.

Kim, K. A., Szatmari, P., Bryson, S. E., Streiner, D. L., & Wilson, F. (2000). The prevalence of anxiety and mood problems among children with autism and Asperger's disorder. *Autism, 4*(2), 117–132.

Klin, A., Pauls, R., Schultz, R., & Volkmar, F. (2005). Three diagnostic approaches to Asperger syndrome: Implication for research. *Journal of Autism and Developmental Disorders, 35*, 221–234.

Klinger, L., & Dawson, G. (1992). Facilitating early social and communicative development in children with autism. In S. Warren & J. Reichle (Eds.), *Causes and effects in communication and language intervention* (pp. 157–186). Baltimore, MD: Paul Brookes.

McCoy, D., Wetherby, A. M., & Woods, J. (2009). *Screening children between 18 and 24 months using the Systematic Observation of Red Flags (SORF) for autism spectrum disorders: A follow-up study.* Presentation at the International Meeting for Autism Research, Chicago, IL.

McEvoy, R. E., Rogers, S. J., & Pennington, B. F. (1993). Executive function and social communication deficits in young autistic children. *Journal of Child Psychology and Psychiatry, 34*, 563–578.

Myles, B. S., Schelvan, R., & Trautman, M. L. (2004). *The hidden curriculum: Practical solutions for understanding unstated rules in social situations.* Shawnee Mission, KS: Autism Asperger Publishing.

Myles, B. S., & Southwick, J. (1999). *Asperger syndrome and difficult moments: Practical solutions for tantrums, rage and meltdowns.* Shawnee Mission, KS: Autism Asperger Publishing.

National Academy Press, Committee on Educational Interventions for Children with Autism, Division of Behavioral and Social Sciences and Education.

National Research Council. (2001). *Educating children with autism.* Washington, DC.

Osterling, J., & Dawson, G. (1994). Early recognition of children with autism: A study of first birthday home videotapes. *Journal of Autism and Developmental Disorders, 24*, 247–257.

Ozonoff, S., & McEvoy, R. E. (1994). A longitudinal study of executive function and theory of mind development in autism. *Development and Psychopathology, 6*, 415–431.

Ozonoff, S., Pennington, B. F., & Rogers, S. J. (1991). Executive function deficits in high-functioning autistic individuals: Relationship to theory of mind. *Journal of Child Psychology and Psychiatry, 32*, 1081–1105.

Prizant, B. M., & Meyer, E. C. (1993). Socioemotional aspects of language and social-communication disorders in young children and their families. *American Journal of Speech-Language Pathology, 2*, 56–71.

Prizant, B. M., Wetherby, A. M., Rubin, E., Laurent, A. C., & Rydell, P. J. (2006). *The SCERTS model: A comprehensive educational approach for children with autism spectrum disorders.* Baltimore, MD: Paul Brookes.

Westby, C. (1988). Children's play: Reflections of social competence. *Seminars in Speech and Language, 9*, 1–13.

Wetherby, A. (2012, January). *DSM V: What does it all mean?* (PowerPoint slides). Keynote address at the 19th annual conference of the Center for Autism and Related Disabilities, Orlando, FL.

Wetherby, A., Woods, J., Allen, L., Cleary, J., Dickinson, H., & Lord, C. (2004). Early indicators of autism spectrum disorders in the second year of life. *Journal of Autism and Developmental Disorders, 34*, 473–493.

Zenko, C. B. (2011). Successfully serving students with ASD in the schools: Let the evidence be your guide. *Perspectives on School Base Issues, 12*(2), 84–90.

2

Understanding Behavior

Introduction

This chapter is not intended to prepare the SLP to provide full behavior analysis services or replace the need for a board-certified behavior analyst (BCBA); however, it is important for the SLP to understand the foundations for common behaviors observed in individuals with ASD. It is the authors' experiences that SLPs often dismiss children with ASD from their caseload secondary to extreme behaviors and difficulty reaching learning targets. Ironically, it is often the communication specialist that is most needed in these situations, as many behaviors are often rooted in fundamental difficulties communicating with people in the child's environment.

This chapter reviews the intricate connections between behavior and all aspects of ASD. It also includes a basic overview of how to analyze behavior and how to use a positive approach to teaching appropriate replacement behavior. As an SLP working with children on the autism spectrum, you *will* encounter *challenging behavior*. The best way to manage challenging behavior is to understand it, understand why it is happening, and understand how to teach a better way to cope or avoid the situation all together.

What Is Behavior?

According to the Merriam-Webster Dictionary (http://www.merriam-webster.com/diction ary/behavior), behavior is defined as:

   a: The manner of conducting oneself.

   b: Anything that an organism does involving action and response to stimulation.

   c: The response of an individual, group, or species to its environment.

In other words, behavior is a way a person acts as a direct result of the stimuli in their environment. SLPs working with children with autism need to understand behavior in a global sense in order to make good clinical decisions and adjustments. Janzen and Zenko (2012) describe behavior in terms of four general concepts (pp. 103–104). First, behavior is communication. All behavior is a response to the current conditions and must be interpreted by others. For children with autism who have limited communication abilities, screaming may be their only way of communicating, "Something is not right!"

Second, behavior is a logical response to the environment where it was first learned. Children with autism often learn best in routines. Sometimes, children on the spectrum incorporate all behaviors that are first learned during a routine whether they were an intentional part of the sequence or not. For example, if you use a therapy ball the first time you see a child with autism, he or she may expect the ball to be in the room every time. The next time the child comes into your room and does not see the ball, he or she may become upset and act out for no apparent reason. In reality, the child is reacting to the absence of the therapy ball (environmental stimulus change) and communicating (via protest), "Where's the ball?"

The third behavioral construct states that behavior is the brain's way of keeping itself stimulated or in equilibrium (Janzen & Zenko, 2012). Children with autism can have a difficult time regulating all of the sensory stimuli bombarding their systems from the environment (Prizant, Wetherby, Rubin, Laurent, & Rydell, 2006). The SCERTS model refers to this as Emotional Regulation (ER). The term emotion is not just referring to feelings but to the overall state of homeostasis or as the authors say "availability to learn" (Prizant et al., 2006, pp. 4–5). Repetitive or stereotypic behaviors (e.g., hand flapping, pacing, rocking, vocalizations, etc.) are often coping mechanisms to help individuals with ASD maintain equilibrium. As human beings, we all have similar coping mechanisms (e.g., chewing gum, drinking caffeine, tapping our feet), but they are usually subtle and easily concealed. As a clinician, it is important to learn what strategies work to help your children with ASD regulate their bodies. The self-regulatory behaviors are not something to get rid of, rather find a way to work around them, incorporate them into the session, or adjust the environment so the child feels more comfortable (See Case Study D–1 on the DVD for a video example).

The last overarching principle regarding behavior is that behavior is an outward expression of an inward state (Janzen & Zenko, 2012). If a person is sick, hungry, tired, anxious, and so forth, their behaviors will reflect it. Individuals who can verbalize their feelings and thoughts can alert others to their altered state. Children on the autism spectrum, who have difficulty communicating, may not be able to verbalize their internal malaise. Therefore, they may act out as their way of communicating something is wrong.

Recognizing the basic human need to express that something is wrong is important when working with students who present challenging behaviors. The behavior you observe may be the child's way of regulating their internal state of turmoil. Prizant et al. (2006) further explain that "children at all developmental stages may exhibit fight-or-flight reactions, which are frequently misinterpreted and treated as behavior problems" (p. 61). Therefore, it is important to remember that behavior always happens for a reason. Becoming a good detective, well-versed in these basic behavior principles, is paramount when providing quality intervention to children with ASD.

Learning Styles, Stress, and Behavior: What's the Connection?

There are some unique learning styles associated with individuals on the autism spectrum. Understanding how ASD affects the way individuals learn, think, and, therefore, respond helps the clinician plan effectively and prepare for unexpected reactions. Figure 2–1 summarizes strengths, personality traits, and deficits commonly associated with ASD. Knowing the strengths of each child helps drive how therapeutic intervention is delivered and received best. Conversely, understanding what things are difficult for children to understand is equally important for the clinician to recognize so their intervention can be adjusted to avoid misunderstanding. Use Figure 2–1 as part of the foundation in the "Balanced Intervention" pyramid (Figure 2–2), "Understanding ASD" and refer back to it often.

Remember, one of the diagnostic features of ASD is the presence of restricted, repetitive, and stereotyped patterns of behaviors, interests, and activities. This manifests in several different ways. Perseverating or *being stuck* on a particular topic, toy, or behavior pattern are a few examples a child may exhibit. Some children have a difficult time accepting any change to their environment or routine and present as a rigid or inflexible thinker. Knowing what behaviors you may see as a result of the child's impairments in the area of restricted or repetitive behaviors and interests can help you prepare your sessions more effectively. One goal of any child on the autism spectrum who has trouble accepting or dealing with change is to teach him or her strategies to use when unexpected events happen. These coping strategies will allow the children with ASD to be more successful in their world that is constantly changing.

> See Case Study C on the DVD for examples of coping strategies (C–3, C–4, C–5, C–7).

Stress plays an intricate part in all human behavior. The definition of the word *stress* varies greatly and often conjures a negative connotation. Selye (1974) states that stress is simply the body's response to demands that are made upon it. There are even differentiating terms for *good* stress—eustress and *bad* stress—distress (Jensen, 1998; Selye, 1974). According to a study by Klinger and Dawson (1992), people have an "optimal level of arousal" that is the result of the right amount of stress. As human beings, we need a certain level of stress to motivate us to accomplish goals; however, too much stress, or distress, can be detrimental (Twachtman-Cullen, 2006). As individuals with ASD have a difficult time regulating their arousal levels and processing all of the environmental or sensory stimuli, they have a smaller window of optimal stress than typically developing, same-aged peers (Klinger & Dawson, 1992). Understanding that individuals with ASD have a narrow window of optimal stress and knowing the warning signs that accompany distress allow the clinician to adjust demands or stressors throughout a therapy session to maximize positive outcomes.

Learning Strengths

The ability to:

- Take in chunks of information quickly—the whole thing
- Remember information for a long time
- Learn to use visual information meaningfully
- Learn and repeat long routines
- Understand and use concrete, context-free information and rules
- Concentrate on narrow topics of specific interest

Personality Traits

The following traits are often associated with individuals who have ASD:

- Perfectionistic
- Righteous
- Honest
- Concrete/literal
- Naïve
- Gullible

Deficits

An inability or decreased ability to automatically, consistently, and/or independently:

- Modulate and process or integrate sensory stimulation
- Control attention, scan to identify, and focus on important information (overfocuses on irrelevant details)
- Analyze, organize, and integrate information to derive meaning (memorizes details, rote responses, and rules rather than concepts)
- Retrieve information in sequential order (interferes with learning cause/effect relationships and ability to predict and prepare for future events)
- Perceive and organize events in time and understand language related to time (leads to confusion and time-related anxiety)
- Understand the complex and changing meanings and nuances of the language (understands and uses the language literally)
- Integrate auditory information efficiently (leads to delays in response time and information gaps)
- Generate alternatives or solve problems that involve hypothesis testing and social judgment (often repeats the same responses over and over)
- Modify or generalize information from one situation to another (learns and uses concepts and skills exactly as taught)
- Control thoughts, movements, and responses (perseverates and gets stuck in motor and verbal routines or responses; may seem driven and compulsive)
- Adjust to new or novel information and events (leads to extreme anxiety associated with change and trying new things)
- Initiate communication to ask for assistance or clarification (leads to confusion, frustration, anxiety, and ineffective behavioral responses)
- Perceive social/cultural rules and the perspective of others (leads to confusion, misunderstandings, and unexpected and ineffective responses)

In summary, individuals with autism are unable to independently integrate bits and pieces of information to make meaning, to expand, or to use information flexibly.

Figure 2–1. Learning strengths, personality traits, and deficits common in autism (Janzen & Zenko, 2012.)

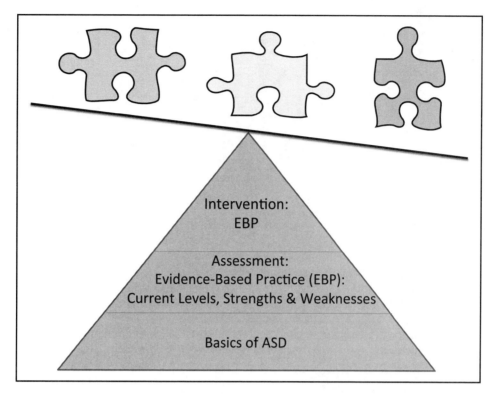

Figure 2–2. Balanced intervention pyramid.

The relation that stress has on behavior is easier to understand in the form of a wave (Janzen, Baron, & Groden, 2006; Janzen & Zenko, 2012). As stressors are introduced, their impact affects the arousal levels of an individual, disrupting the ideal level of homeostasis. The bottom of the wave represents the calm of equilibrium or the optimal arousal level. As stressors are introduced, the wave starts to build, responses to the stressors become apparent and continue to rise as the arousal level heightens (Janzen et al., 2006; Janzen & Zenko, 2012). The wave crests at maximum stress levels with behaviors that typically mirror a fight-or-flight reaction. As the stressors are reduced and the person begins to feel the immediate threat or danger is over, the individual's arousal levels begin to come back down toward equilibrium (Janzen et al., 2006; Janzen & Zenko, 2012).

The speed at which this stress curve climbs or falls and the height of the peak all depend on the timing and appropriate intervention strategies of the interventionist. Recognizing the warning signs that the individual with ASD is feeling distress and diffusing or removing the stressors is the best way of preventing the wave from cresting. If the warning signs are missed or handled poorly and the behavior peaks, the only course of action is to solve the problem quickly while keeping everyone safe and encouraging relaxation (Janzen et al., 2006; Janzen & Zenko, 2012). This is *not a teachable moment,* so any attempts to discuss the situation, reprimand, and so forth, will only make things worse. As the individual starts to calm down and return to equilibrium, this downward crest is a delicate state that needs to focus on relaxation and not rehashing what just happened. Figure 2–3 outlines the profile of stress, behavior, and intervention appropriate for each phase of the stress curve.

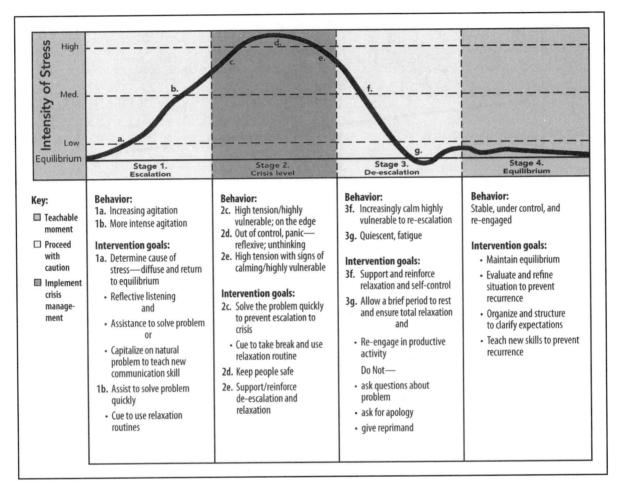

Figure 2–3. Profile of stress and corresponding interventions (Modified from Janzen & Zenko, 2012).

Positive Behavior Support (PBS): What All SLPs Need to Know

According to the Association for Positive Behavior Support (2012), Positive Behavior Support (PBS) is "a set of research-based strategies used to increase the quality of life and decrease the problem behavior by teaching new skills and making changes to a person's environment" (http://www.apbs.org/new_apbs/genIntro.aspx). There are several facets of the PBS approach, but the one SLPs need to understand and use the most is functional behavioral assessment (FBA). FBA provides a systematic way to dissect behavior starting with a concrete description of the behavior, what happened just before and after the behavior occurred, and creating hypotheses based on the observation data regarding the possible function of the behavior (Association for Positive Behavior Support, 2012; Carr et al., 2002). Most FBA utilize the Antecedent, Behavior, Consequence (ABC) format of data collection to create hypotheses surrounding why the behavior is occurring. These data, collected on a simple ABC charting form, helps the team brainstorm possible replacement behaviors that are more acceptable by all parties (Carr et al., 2002).

For sample data tracking charts and other user-friendly PBS tools, go to http://www.pbis.org

PBS strives to find a positive solution to challenging behavior by creating data-driven hypotheses to answer the question, "Why is he or she doing that?" to create and teach the individual replacement behaviors that will serve the same function as the challenging behavior.

SLPs who work with individuals with ASD need to know how to collect ABC data. Recognizing the antecedents, or what happened right before a behavior is observed, requires the SLP to recall how characteristics of ASD and the effect of stress on behavior may affect the antecedent. Figure 2–4 lists six questions to ask when trying to determine the possible cause or antecedent of a challenging behavior. These questions help the clinician keep the underlying effects of ASD in mind when trying to interpret challenging behavior.

Behavior Strategies That Work

According to the National Autism Center's National Standards Report (2009), interventions involving antecedent alterations to improve behavior and interventions that used the basic principles of PBS have enough empirical support to be considered *established* evidence based practice. In the 330 studies, the National Autism Center's report reviewed that out of both of the general behavioral approaches listed above, several effective strategies and techniques were listed that can be applied in the speech and language setting.

For the complete report, go to
http://www.nationalautismcenter.org/nsp

Using visual supports to increase understanding, predictability, and, therefore, reduce anxiety is one strategy that proved effective. In a clinical setting, creating a visual schedule of each session is one way to apply this concept (see Figure 2–5 for an example). Visual schedules help reduce anxiety by increasing the predictability of what to expect and can also be used as a form of priming. Priming involves reviewing a topic before it is actually presented, so the individual can prepare before instruction begins.

See Case Study D-1 through D-5 on the DVD for examples of how a visual schedule can help reduce anxiety.

Another way to utilize visual supports is to create a First/Then board where you depict a less-preferred activity in the first column—one that the child can do quickly and success-

The following six questions can be committed to memory and used as a quick mental checklist when a behavior signals a problem. These questions address the common learning styles, deficits, and unique needs of people on the autism spectrum.

1. What is new, changed, or missing (related to people, time, space, or events)?

2. What may have been misinterpreted or misunderstood?
   - The directions? Directions directed to others nearby?
   - A conversation? A conversation between others in another area?
   - Something read in the daily paper or a magazine?
   - Something heard on radio or TV?
   - A word? A concept? A rule?

3. Is some element of the instructional plan or task unclear? For example, does the individual really understand (is it visually clear):
   - What to do? Both sides of the picture—what can and cannot be done?
   - Why it is being done (the meaning, outcome, or purpose)?
   - How and where to do it?
   - Where to start? When to start?
   - What materials, people, or equipment are needed?
   - When it is finished?
   - What to do next?
   - When a favorite activity or interaction is scheduled?
   - When help or clarification is needed?

4. Is it a specific communication problem? Does the learner have an effective way to spontaneously:
   - Ask for help or clarification?
   - Get out of a boring or disliked situation?
   - Start or end an interaction?
   - Get a break, relief from overstimulation?
   - Specify choices? Needs?

5. Is some element of the environment confusing, irritating, disrupting or overwhelming (e.g., heat, light, noise, textures, crowding, arrangement of materials, work too difficult, a medical problem)?

6. Is boredom or lack of stimulation the issue?

Figure 2–4. Checklist to identify potential reasons for "challenging behaviors" (Janzen & Zenko, 2012).

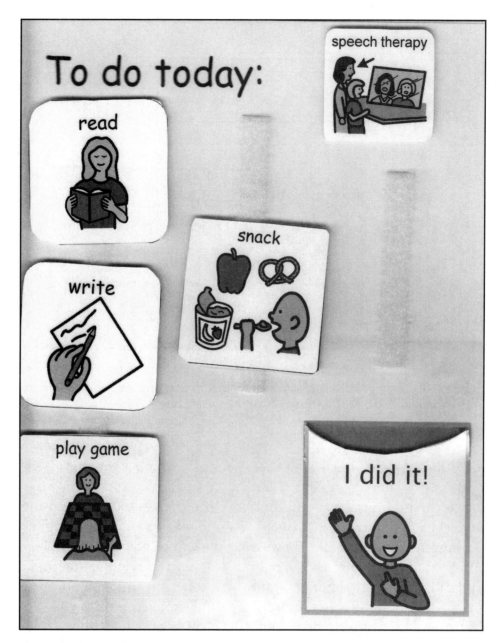

Figure 2–5. Sample visual schedule created by the University of Florida Center for Autism and Related Disabilities using Boardmaker software.

fully so you can move on to the more-preferred activity, shown in the then column. This teaches the Premack principle: People are more likely to complete a less desired activity if it is immediately followed by a highly desired object or activity (Premack & Collier, 1962). See Figure 2–6 for an example of a First-Then board used by a school-age child.

See http://www.sage-ereference.com/view/cbt/n2094.xml for a more detailed explanation of the Premack principle.

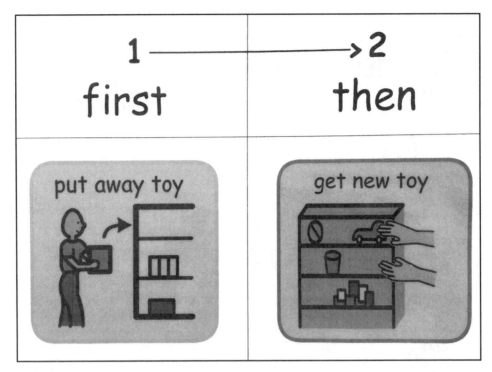

Figure 2–6. Sample first/then board created by the University of Florida Center for Autism and Related Disabilities using Boardmaker software.

Utilizing visual supports to create a choice board is another way to increase communication and decrease the probability of challenging behaviors. Allowing individuals the opportunity to choose what they want and have the choices in an easy communicative format (visuals) helps improve positive behavior and outcomes, while providing a natural reason to communicate. Figure 2–7 shows a simple choice board that can be adapted to use in multiple situations. Children can help create the visuals or pictures that go on their choice boards, thus providing another naturalistic communication building opportunity. (See files on the DVD for multiple examples of visual supports and how they are used).

Finding ways to motivate children with ASD is often difficult. Using specific, positive praise and incorporating a token economy system of positive reinforcement, utilizing meaningful tokens, is effective (National Autism Center, 2009) (see Figure 2–8 for an example). Another way to increase motivation and participation is by following the child's lead and incorporating his or her special interest areas into actual therapy sessions (Sussman, 1999). If you use their special interest areas, you are more likely to get and keep their attention, therefore, increasing your quality interaction or intervention time.

Utilizing the fair pair concept (White & Haring, 1976) is another proven behavioral strategy. The fair pair concept basically states that if you tell a child, "No, don't do _____" you must automatically follow up with a "Yes, you can do _____ instead." Children with ASD do not always know the proper or "OK" thing to do if you only tell them what they cannot do. If you follow the fair pair rule, you can prevent more undesired behavior by simply telling and showing the children what they can and should do instead. For

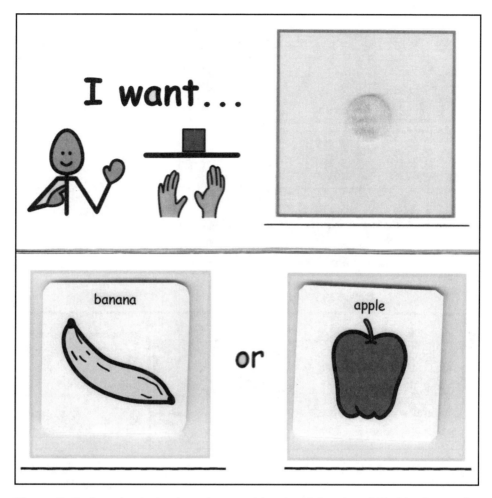

Figure 2–7. Sample choice board created by the University of Florida Center for Autism and Related Disabilities using Boardmaker software.

example, if I say, "Don't run." I need to follow up that statement with "I need you to walk." Creating visuals that go along with each fair pair is also helpful. Creating visual fair pair charts can be an activity you do with the child in therapy to provide an active learning component to each fair pair. (see Figure 2–9 for an example of a visual fair pair.)

Knowing When to Refer or Ask for Help

There comes a time in every clinician's career when he or she has tried all the strategies covered in this chapter and more, but nothing seems to be working. The SLP cannot deliver effective intervention because the child's behavior is interfering. One suggestion is to video tape a session so the clinician can step back and try and see potential antecedents that he or she could not see while in the moment. Asking a colleague to view the tape and share ideas is another way to try and understand why the behaviors are happening and how to best address them.

If the child's behavior continues to interfere with intervention, consult with a BCBA who specializes in ASD. Bringing in a colleague with specific training, knowledge, and experience in behavior analysis is a common practice when working with children on

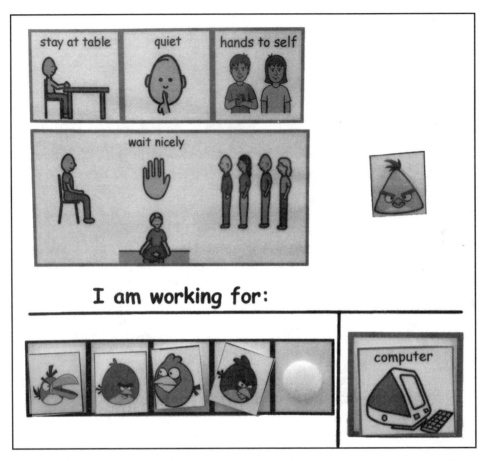

Figure 2–8. Sample token reinforcement system using a child's interest in Angry Birds as tokens created by the University of Florida Center for Autism and Related Disabilities using Boardmaker software and Google images.

the autism spectrum. Ask the family if they are already working with a BCBA and if so, contact that person and ask him or her to collaborate. Asking a family what other professionals they are already working with when you first meet them is a good idea so you can start working as a team from the beginning. Collaborating with all the professionals on a child's intervention team (for example, a BCBA) allows the SLP to incorporate the same strategies and vocabulary the child is already using with other professionals.

Summary

One of the hardest things about working with children on the autism spectrum who have challenging behaviors is remembering they are not doing this on purpose to punish you. However, in the heat of the moment, it often feels this way. The behavior you are seeing is a result of something in the environment that is not making sense to the child on the spectrum. Go back to what you know about ASD, how it affects the learning styles, and what role stress plays in behavior. Try to see the world through the eyes of the child with autism and make sense of what his or her behavior is trying to tell you. Analyze the

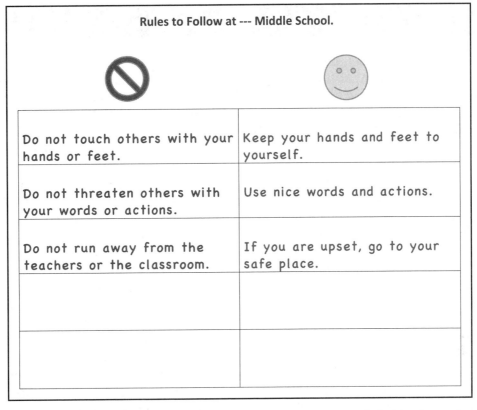

Figure 2–9. Sample fair pair visual created by the University of Florida Center for Autism and Related Disabilities using Microsoft Word.

behavior using the ABC format. Look at the behavior from a scientific perspective and go back to the four principles of behavior discussed at the beginning of the chapter. Behavior, by definition, is a reaction to the stimuli in the environment. In a clinical setting, the clinician is part of the environment. Therefore, if you want a child's behavior to change, you may need to change your own behavior. Always remember the old saying, an ounce of prevention is worth a pound of cure, so take the time to try and identify the antecedents, focus your time on adjusting the antecedents, and teach positive alternative behaviors.

Learning Tool

1. What are the four principals of behavior discussed in this chapter, and how do they relate to a clinical setting?

2. Explain how sensory challenges affect the behavior of children on the autism spectrum.

3. What are three effective strategies a clinician can do to address challenging behaviors exhibited by children on the autism spectrum?

References

Association for Positive Behavior Support. (2012). What is PBS? Retrieved from http://www.apbs.org/new_apbs/genIntro.aspx

Carr, E. G., Dunlap, G., Horner, R. H., Koegel, R. L., Turnbull, A., Sailor, W., . . . Fox, L. (2002). *Journal of Positive Behavior Interventions, 4*(1), 4–16.

Janzen, J. E., Baron, M. G., & Groden, J. (2006). In M. G. Baron, J. Groden, G. Groden, & L. P. Lipsitt (Eds.), *Stress and coping in autism* (pp. 324–350). Oxford, UK: Oxford University Press.

Janzen, J. E., & Zenko, C. B. (2012). *Understanding the nature of autism: A guidebook to the autism spectrum disorders* (3rd ed.). San Antonio, TX: Hammill Institute on Disabilities.

Jensen, E. (1998). *Teaching the brain in mind.* Alexandria, VA: Association for Supervision and Curriculum Development.

Klinger, L., & Dawson, G. (1992). Facilitating early social and communicative development in children with autism. In S. Warren & J. Reichle (Eds.), *Causes and effects in communication and language intervention* (pp. 157–186). Baltimore, MD: Paul Brookes.

National Autism Center. (2009). *National standards report: The national standards project—addressing the need for evidence-based practice guidelines for autism spectrum disorders.* Randolph, MA: National Autism Center.

Premack, D., & Collier, G. (1962). Analysis of nonreinforcement variable affecting response probability. *Psychological Monographs: General and Applied, 76,* 5.

Prizant, B. M., Wetherby, A. M., Rubin, E., Laurent, A. C., & Rydell, P. J. (2006). *The SCERTS model: A comprehensive educational approach for children with autism spectrum disorders.* Baltimore, MD: Paul Brookes.

Selye, H. (1974). *Stress without distress.* Philadelphia, PA: Lippincott.

Sussman, F. (1999). *More than words: A guide to helping parents promote communication and social skills in children with autism spectrum disorder.* Toronto, Canada: The Hanen Centre.

Twachtman-Cullen, D. (2006). Communication and stress in students with autism spectrum disorder. In M. G. Baron, J. Groden, G. Groden, & L. P. Lipsitt (Eds.), *Stress and coping in autism* (pp. 302–323). Oxford, UK: Oxford University Press.

White, O. R., & Haring, N. G. (1976). *Exceptional teaching: A multimedia training package.* Columbus, OH: Merrill.

CHAPTER

3

Assessment

Introduction

The goal of this book is to assist SLPs with designing a balanced intervention program for working with children with ASD. The journey to building a balanced intervention program begins with a comprehensive assessment of baseline functioning, or present level, across areas related to social communication. This assessment, paired with knowledge of evidence-based practice, serves as a road map to help identify which routes need to be taken to help the child with ASD reach successful outcomes.

SLPs are involved in the diagnostic process of individuals with ASDs in multiple ways. First, many SLPs will participate on a diagnostic team composed of many medical and/ or educational professionals determining whether or not a child has ASD. As discussed previously, the diagnosis of ASD requires observations of difficulties in the area of social communication and restricted, repetitive and stereotypic behaviors and interests. SLPs are a valuable resource on the evaluation team, providing the clinical expertise needed to quantify and describe the nature of the social communicative deficit. The SLP often has children with previous diagnoses of ASD referred to him or her to assist with further assessment of the specific social communication difficulties that need to be targeted in therapy. SLPs may also find themselves evaluating a child who has not yet been diagnosed with ASD, but is demonstrating red flags associated with having ASD. The communication assessment provided by an SLP is a valuable tool to: assist a team with evaluation of social communication as part of the process of diagnosing ASD, provide an accurate profile of the child's social communication, provide a description of the child's presenting communication skills, and identify areas of concern. The assessment may lead to a referral to a diagnostic team that can make the diagnosis of ASD if appropriate.

Early Identification

The National Research Council (2001) noted "the diagnosis of autism can be made reliably in 2 year olds by professionals experienced in the diagnostic assessment of young children with autism spectrum disorders" (p. 212). Earlier diagnosis of ASD, and thus an earlier provision of intervention, has been associated with increased outcomes (National Research Council, 2001). For this reason, it is imperative that professionals are prepared to give formal diagnoses when appropriate so that children can have access to services as early as possible (National Research Council, 2001). Professionals from multiple disciplines, including speech language pathology, are currently researching improved ways to identify children with ASD at even younger ages. An excellent resource for clinicians is the ASD Video Glossary, which shows video clips comparing children with and without ASD.

To view the ASD video glossary, go to
http://www.autismspeaks.org/what-autism/video-glossary.

The American Academy of Pediatrics recommends developmental surveillance be incorporated for all children at every well-child preventive care visit, with screening for developmental delays occurring at 9-, 18-, and 24- or 30-month well visits. The American Academy of Pediatrics also recommends that all children should be routinely screened for ASD specifically at 18 and 24 months of age. There are many screening tools that can be used by medical professionals to assist with the early identification of children with ASD. The Centers for Disease Control and Prevention (2012) recommended that "further developmental evaluation is required whenever a child fails to meet any of the following milestones:

- Babbling by 12 months;
- Gesturing (e.g., pointing, waving bye-bye) by 12 months;
- Single words by 16 months;
- Two-word spontaneous (not just echolalic) phrases by 24 months;
- Loss of any language or social skills at any age."

See the following link for full document
http://www.cdc.gov/ncbddd/autism/hcp-recommendations.html.

When looking at this list of developmental milestones considered to be red flags for ASD, it is easy to see how the SLP might be involved early in the diagnostic process and facilitate early identification.

The Communication and Symbolic Behavior Scales Developmental Profile Infant-Toddler Checklist (CSBS-DP Infant-Toddler Checklist; Wetherby & Prizant, 2002) is one tool to screen for possible communication delays in young children, ages 6 to 24 months of age. Screening tools specifically designed to identify ASD include the Modified Checklist for Autism in Toddlers (M-CHAT; Robbins, Fein, & Barton, 1999) and the Screening Tool for Autism in Two-Year-Olds (STAT; Stone & Ousley, 2004). For older children or children who are on the mild end of the spectrum, the Social Communication Questionnaire (SCQ; Rutter, Bailey, Berument, Lord, & Pickles, 2003) or the Autism Spectrum Screening Questionnaire (ASSQ; Ehlers, Gillberg, & Wing, 1999) are often used as screening tools.

The following links have information about ASD screening tools and recommendations and procedures:

http://www.cdc.gov/ncbddd/autism/hcp-screening.html

https://www.firstsigns.org/screening/tools/rec.htm

http://www.nimh.nih.gov/health/publications/a-parents-guide-to-autism-spectrum-disorder/complete-index.shtml

http://firstwords.fsu.edu/index.php/autism-spectrum-disorders/22-redflags

http://firstwords.fsu.edu/pdf/checklist.pdf (CSBS-DP Infant-Toddler Checklist)

http://www2.gsu.edu/~psydlr/Diana_L._Robins,_Ph.D.html (M-CHAT)

http://stat.vueinnovations.com/ (STAT)

The SLP often serves as one of the first responders in the effort to identify children with ASD. Among parents' earliest concerns is often their child's decreased nonverbal or verbal communication, difficulty in interactions with peers, and/or presence of problem behaviors, which is often related to the child's communication difficulties.

At a recent seminar on ASD, a parent spoke about her family's path to getting a diagnosis for their child. After speaking with their pediatrician, the child was referred to an SLP. The child initially received services from an SLP because the child was not yet talking and was not using a variety of speech sounds. Prior to the age of four, the child was diagnosed with childhood apraxia of speech, as well as receptive and expressive language disorders. The SLP was the first to document the difficulties in the areas of social communication, including joint attention and social reciprocity. The SLP referred the family to a local psychologist and collaborated with the professional to assist with the evaluation process leading to the ultimate diagnosis of Pervasive Developmental Disorder-Not Otherwise Specified (PDD-NOS). The parent spoke about how the SLP was the key person that led to her child being diagnosed due to the SLP's specialty in the area of communication. The SLP was able to provide helpful information regarding red flags for ASD that helped the parents understand the importance of and reason for the referral to other professionals. The SLP also provided the profile of social communication skills necessary for the medical team to appropriately provide a diagnosis for the child. This diagnosis led to increased support and interventions for the child, who is successfully participating in general education with support today.

Understanding Multidisciplinary Assessments

Once a screening tool is administered resulting in concerns, a systematic evaluation is required to make an ASD diagnosis. Ideally, multiple disciplines are involved in the comprehensive evaluation process to determine if the child has ASD. Although the American Speech-Language-Hearing Association (2006) states that an SLP can make a diagnosis of ASD if they have significant experience working with this population, the American Speech-Language-Hearing Association also states that an ASD diagnosis is typically given by a team of people, including an SLP, who have all conducted various assessments. Other professionals most likely to be on a diagnostic team are: physicians, clinical or school psychologists, educators, occupational therapists (OTs), physical therapists (PTs), and nurses (American Speech-Language-Hearing Association, 2006; National Research Council, 2001).

Remember, an ASD diagnosis is based on direct observations and information collected from the people who know the child; there is no specific medical test, bloodwork, and so forth that can diagnose autism. Therefore, the few standardized measures used specifically to diagnose ASD are based on observations and interviews. The two gold-standard tests used to diagnose ASD and to define ASD for research purposes are the *Autism Diagnostic Observation Schedule-Second Edition-ADOS-2* (Lord et al., 2012) and the *Autism Diagnostic Interview–Revised-ADI–R* (Rutter, Le Couteur, & Lord, 2003). Both the *ADOS-2* and the *ADI-R* require additional training to be qualified to administer the test. An SLP can be the professional who administers these tests if they complete the proper training. Regardless of whether or not the SLP receives *ADOS-2* or *ADI-R* training, it is important to be able to read and understand the results of each test to create meaningful intervention plans.

Two other standardized measures frequently used to diagnose ASD are the *Childhood Autism Rating Scale-Second Edition-CARS-2* (Schopler, Van Bourgondien, Wellman, & Love, 2010) and the *Gilliam Autism Rating Scale-Second Edition-GARS-2* (Gilliam, 2006). These tests do not require specialized training for professionals who administer them, so in theory, an SLP could administer either test. However, physicians, psychologists, and/or educators are more likely to give the *CARS-2* or the *GARS-2* during a diagnostic evaluation. Again, as an SLP working with children on the autism spectrum, it is not imperative that you know how to administer these diagnostic tests, but it is important for you to understand the results and how they relate to intervention needs.

Assessment of Children with ASD: General Considerations

Children with ASD present with a scattered profile of skills and difficulties (Klin, Saulnier, Tsatsanis, & Volkmar, 2005). This profile is best represented by a description of areas of skills and deficits rather than an overall average number describing global performance. Klin et al. (2005) stated, "It is important to delineate a profile of assets and deficits rather than simply presenting an overall and often misleading summary score or measure because such global scores may represent the averaging of highly discrepant skills" (p. 775). Similarly, children with ASD often have areas of specific interest and may possess extensive knowledge on these topics (e.g., letters/numbers, mechanical and physical engineering concepts, etc.). These areas of increased knowledge might skew the overall performance on some measures (e.g., children may have "splinter skills" such as precocious decoding skills, visuospatial skills, etc.) and misrepresent the child's true learning and adaptive functioning skills across all areas (Klin et al., 2005; National Research Council, 2001). Additionally, it is important for the clinician to understand that one single assessment instrument will not likely provide sufficient information needed for a comprehensive communication evaluation (Lord & Corsello, 2005). Use of a variety of assessments and/or modifying test formats for dynamic assessments will yield the most comprehensive information (Klin et al., 2005; National Research Council, 2001). Choosing the right battery of assessment tools is a complex decision dependent on several factors, including the child's level of verbal communication, attention and speed of processing, tolerance of new transitions, and ability to respond to verbal instructions and social expectations (National Research Council, 2001). The choice in assessment tools will also be dependent on the examiner's goals for the evaluation or assessment: qualification for educational services, medical diagnosis resulting in third-party payment for intervention services, intervention planning, progress monitoring, or re-evaluation. The following section provides a comparison of differing types of assessments and their clinical uses and limitations.

Types of Measures Used in Assessment with Children with ASD

Norm-Referenced Measures

Norm-referenced assessments are standardized to compare an individual's performance to that of a larger, normative group (Shipley & McAfee, 2004). By definition, standardized tests provide a *standard* or set way to administer or score the test, which allows for comparison with a normal distribution (Paul, 2007). The quantitative results achieved, such as standard scores and percentile ranks, allow the clinician to determine if skills fall within or outside of the normal range of variation in skills (Paul, 2007).

Benefits of use: Norm-referenced measures are best used in evaluations, or in determining initial or continued eligibility for services. Insurance companies and school districts typically prefer standardized test results when possible in order to qualify a child for services (Shipley & McAfee, 2004). Norm-referenced measures provide clear guidelines for administration and interpretation to assist the clinician and, therefore, are considered to have increased objectivity. They are particularly helpful when the clinician is initially evaluating a child and seeks to learn if certain skills fall within the normal range or if a disorder exists (Paul, 2007). When used carefully, some standardized measures might help to quantify individual skills within the child's profile of strengths and weaknesses.

Limitations: Children with ASD often have difficulty with standardized assessment procedures due to difficulties with following verbally mediated instructions and social reinforcement (National Research Council, 2001). Standardized assessments have specific rules regarding testing format and by definition do not allow for individualization of the test administration (Paul, 2007; Shipley & McAfee, 2004). Each question or testing section may have set ways of delivering questions or instructions with little variability in terms of cues and prompts permitted. Additionally, norm-referenced tests measure isolated skills without looking at influencing factors, and the format is out of context from a true communicative situation (Shipley & McAfee, 2004). For example, one item on the Pragmatic Judgment subtest of the Comprehensive Assessment of Spoken Language (CASL; Carrow-Woolfolk, 2008) asks, "Suppose the telephone rings. You pick it up. What do you say?" This context is theoretical and may yield different results depending on if the child was handed a real, ringing phone and told to answer it. These contexts (e.g., in the previous example, at home answering a phone) often change rapidly between each question or subtest, requiring frequent attention shifting. Children with ASD are known to have difficulty with shifting attention, which makes performance in these conditions difficult. Formal testing procedures are often difficult for children with ASD to understand, and their performance in these situations may not represent their true adaptive functioning (i.e., ability to translate skills to use in real-life contexts) in everyday life (National Research Council, 2001). "Because formal assessment tools may not accurately detect problems in the social use of language and communication, eligibility may need to be based on clinical judgment and more informal, observational measures" (American

Speech-Language-Hearing Association, 2006). Therefore, standardized assessments should represent only one part of a comprehensive communication evaluation for children with ASD (Klin et al., 2005; Paul, 2005).

Cindy, a 5-year-old preschool child transitioning into kindergarten in the next year, had previously been given the *Preschool Language Scales-Fifth Edition* (*PLS-5*; Zimmerman, Steiner, & Pond, 2011) during her initial communication evaluation. This test provides an overall standard score for auditory comprehension and for expressive language, as well as a total language score. Cindy's global language scores all fell more than two standard deviations below the mean, which initially assisted with her qualification for exceptional student education (ESE) in a full-time, school-based program. It was noted that the global language measure provided an average of skills, with her significantly decreased oral language blending with her area of strength, early literacy skills. This lead to a summary score that did not truly convey an accurate profile of her skills across linguistic areas. At the time of her reevaluation, the school-based team was considering her profile of skills to determine her placement for the next year. The clinician decided to administer a wide variety of measures to show the variability in her profile: both her strengths and areas in need of intervention. In terms of standardized assessments, an updated global language measure, the *Clinical Evaluation of Language Fundamentals Preschool-Second Edition* (*CELF-P2*; Wiig, Secord, & Semel, 2006) was administered to provide information across a broad range of linguistic skills: semantics, syntax, morphology, phonology, and pragmatics. Results of this measure continued to yield overall skills more than one and a half standard deviations below the mean and confirmed the child continued to need ESE services. The *Receptive One-Word Picture Vocabulary Test-Fourth Edition* (*ROWPVT-4*; Martin & Brownell, 2011), a single-word receptive vocabulary measure, was also administered that revealed skills within the normal range. A test of early literacy skills, the *Test of Early Reading Ability-Third Edition* (*TERA-3*; Reid, Hrasko, & Hammill, 2001) also yielded results above the normal range, due to her letter, number, sound/letter correspondence knowledge, and her precocious abilities to decode text. The various standardized measures administered helped the examiner demonstrate for the educational team that although overall language skills were significantly decreased, as noted on the *PLS-5* and *CELF-P2* administrations, there were areas of significant strengths and an overall wide range in skills across all areas. The discrepancy in results of the global language measure (*CELF-P2*) versus the single-word vocabulary assessment (*ROWPVT-4*) was consistent with parent and teacher observations that although Cindy seems to know about many of the concepts covered in the classroom, she has significant difficulty with listening in the classroom and relaying what she knows. She demonstrated a particular strength in the area of emergent literacy development, as shown on the *TERA-3*, which was consistent with parent and preschool teacher reports. Listening skills and expression were difficult due to continued deficits in listening comprehension and expression for sentence and discourse level language. Further evaluation of semantics, syntax, morphology, and pragmatics was conducted using alternate test formats. See below for descriptions of additional types of assessments.

Criterion-Referenced Measures

Criterion-referenced measures provide a comparison of individual performance to a set "expected level of performance" (Shipley & McAfee, 2004, p. 10). The results reveal whether or not the individual meets a designated level of expectation for a particular skill, as opposed to norm-referenced, which compares a child's performance with other children's performance (Paul, 2007; Ruscello, 2001). The assessment can be standardized or nonstandardized (Shipley & McAfee, 2004). An example of a criterion-referenced measure designed for use with children with ASD is the SCERTS Assessment Process (SAP) described within the SCERTS model (Prizant, Wetherby, Rubin, Laurent, & Rydell, 2006). The SAP lets the examiner compare the child's performance across the targeted areas (social communication and emotional regulation) and compare with developmental expectations based on known research (Prizant et al., 2006). The SAP is also curriculum-based, in that the assessment process allows the clinician to determine where the child's skill level falls based on the associated curricular sequence found in the SCERTS model curriculum (Prizant et al., 2006).

Benefits of use: Criterion-referenced measures typically provide guidance for administration and interpretation to assist the clinician and, therefore, are considered to have increased objectivity (Shipley & McAfee, 2004). These measures may also be sufficient for use in qualification for services or gaining third-party payment, although norm-referenced measures may be required for initial diagnosis purposes (Paul, 2007). When the criterion-referenced measure is not standardized, it allows for some individualization in administration, which may be significantly helpful when assessing individuals with ASD.

The nonstandardized criterion-referenced measure offers the opportunity for looking at specific communication skills, while still allowing for flexibility in administration (Paul, 2007). This allows the examiner to compare performance with developmental criteria while still providing some adaptation for individual support needs. Criterion-referenced measures may be particularly helpful for monitoring progress in intervention and to assist with intervention planning (Paul, 2007).

Limitations: If the criterion-referenced measure is standardized, then typically there will be precise rules for administration and interpretation. Thus, the same limitations would apply for criterion-referenced measures as compared with norm-referenced measures. Like norm-referenced measures discussed previously, criterion-referenced assessments target isolated skills in a format that is out of context from a real-life communicative situation (Shipley & McAfee, 2004). See the discussion above regarding limitations of norm-referenced measures due to these factors.

During the latter half of her kindergarten year, our case example, Cindy, was displaying difficulty with reading comprehension. Both the parent and the teacher reported that while Cindy read the words of the stories fluently, she seemed to have very little grasp of the details and had difficulty answering basic questions about the text. The parent and teacher approached the clinician about helping to determine the extent of Cindy's difficulty and to assist with remediation. The clinician suspected the child's language comprehension difficulties were at the root, noting that Cindy had difficulty answering "wh" questions in general. The *Qualitative Reading Inventory-Fifth Edition* (QRI-5; Leslie & Caldwell, 2011) was administered to assess her single-word reading level, reading accuracy, and reading comprehension. The *QRI-5* provides a criterion rating of "independent, instructional, or frustration" for each aspect of reading (i.e., single-word reading, reading accuracy, reading comprehension). Cindy was noted to read both single words and connected text (reading accuracy) independently at a first-grade level. In contrast, her reading comprehension at the first-grade level was at "frustration." Cindy had difficulty comprehending the language of the text and was noted to have difficulty with questions that were not represented in a picture within the story. Additionally, the clinician noted frequent confusion of the "wh" questions, even early forms that had been previously learned in therapy. The results of this assessment provided valuable information regarding how Cindy was applying learned language comprehension skills to written language and thus pointing the direction for future intervention needs.

Authentic Assessments, Including Observational Assessments and Caregiver Checklists

Authentic assessments provide information about what an individual does or does not do in various real-life situations. The examiner only provides enough structure to elicit the targeted skills. For example, to elicit information about the child's ability to request needs and wants, the clinician might observe communication skills during snack time within the classroom, being sure that the child was not given all snack items at once without communicating. This type of assessment also can be conducted over time to provide information about performance across multiple settings, with differing levels of novelty, and while interacting with various individuals involved (e.g., parents, teachers, intervention professionals, etc.). Examples of authentic assessments that might be utilized in a communication evaluation for a child with ASD (adapted from Shipley & McAfee, 2004):

- Language sampling
- Speech sampling
- Checklists (developmental, curricular)
- Caregiver and teacher checklists, interviews
- Play analysis through structured symbolic, social play situations.

Benefits of use: Because of a lack of predetermined administration procedures, authentic assessment allows for the greatest amount of flexibility and individualization (Shipley & McAfee, 2004). This is especially important when assessing children who are typically not represented in normative samples such as children who utilize augmentative or alternative communication (AAC) or come from culturally and linguistically diverse backgrounds. Children with ASD often present with widely varied skills across different situations (National Research Council, 2001). Some aspects of the setting that may influence the child's performance include "novelty, degree of structure provided, and complexity of the environment" (National Research Council, 2001, p. 27). As stated previously, authentic assessments allow for multiple sources of qualitative information, including the child's communication performance across people, environments, and levels of novelty and support. Authentic assessment allows evaluation of the child's true communicative functioning in real-life contexts, rather than assessing pragmatic language just at the knowledge level (Bellini, 2006).

Authentic assessments also can provide valuable qualitative information regarding types of supports that assist the child which is an important tool for therapy planning. For example, the clinician might observe that when the child is verbally asked which beverage she would like with her lunch, she does not answer. However, when the caregiver asks the question and holds up two choices, the child completes the communicative act and verbally tells the caregiver which beverage she chooses. Overall, the authentic assessment provides the most valuable information for intervention planning.

Assessments that allow for structured reports of parental or teacher's observations also provide valuable information to the SLP. Because it is important to gain insight into the child's profile of skills across multiple people and environments, parent/teacher observations provide valuable information that might otherwise be difficult to attain. This is particularly true for obtaining information about social functioning across widely varying contexts, such as with highly familiar people (e.g., parents, grandparents, siblings, etc.) versus group settings with peers.

Limitations: Authentic assessment provides a qualitative analysis of the client's performance, which takes more specialized skill from the clinician. Novice clinicians may have difficulty providing authentic assessment due to decreased experience. This approach does not provide a predetermined sequence of tasks or readily available materials, so it requires increased planning time. Authentic assessments are not structured, known test formats, such as those found with norm-referenced and criterion-referenced measures, which is contrary to what is preferred by insurance companies and school districts when determining qualification for educational services or third-party payment.

> To gain information about Cindy's communication skills in a natural context, the clinician observed Cindy within her classroom and collected a conversational language sample. The sample revealed Cindy frequently used delayed, immediate, and mitigated echolalia functionally to respond and participate with peers and adults. The observation also revealed that Cindy had more difficulty with interactions with peers as compared with adults. She was not observed to initiate communication frequently, but did typically respond to communication bids from adults. Often, adults had to repeat their questions or comments directed toward Cindy so that she would answer. Cindy's peers were noted to abandon their attempts rather than repair the communication, resulting in fewer conversational interractions with peers. A social communication or social skills checklist was completed based on the observation, specifically the *Assessment of Social and Communication Skills for Children with Autism* (Quill, 2000). The checklist guided the clinician's observations, revealing concerns in the area of conversational skills, including turn taking, topic maintenance, joint attention with the speaker, and so forth. This information, paired with the standardized evaluation results, provided a well-rounded profile of Cindy's pattern of strengths and areas of difficulty and assisted with developing her future intervention plan.

Assessment Procedures: Prepare for Success

The SLP should keep in mind what has been previously described regarding the different learning and behavioral profiles associated with individuals with an ASD. This knowledge will help the SLP prepare for evaluations and ongoing assessments with children with ASD in ways that will bring maximum success. The following are important considerations to make when preparing for an assessment with an individual that presents with or is suspected of having an ASD.

Before the Assessment

> During a play assessment, the clinician noted Cindy played with the pretend kitchen and play food presented. The clinician noted that Cindy had an established routine with the toys, pretending to be a chef. She methodically asked the clinician, "What food do you want?," cooked the food in the toy frying pan, and then put it on a plate in front of the clinician. She rarely referenced the clinician's face and did not respond to the clinician's verbal attempts to participate in the play. At one point, Cindy took the toy frying pan and went to the therapy room mirror. She held it with both hands next to her head, saying, "Who are you?" with a big smile. The clinician was unsure what this aside was in reference to and suspected it was delayed echolalia of a favored television show or movie. Afterward, the clinician verified with the mother that the child had been repeating a line from one of her favorite Disney movies, *Tangled* (2010), where Rapunzel uses a frying pan to defend herself. The child's mother also informed the clinician that Cindy always played chef in this exact way and that she had been taught this sequence with a previous therapist.

The above case provides an example of how children with ASD may present with different skills compared with what is expected from typically developing children. In order to best prepare for an evaluation with a child with ASD, there are many things the clinician can do to help with interpreting what skills the child does and does not present with. See the following list adapted from Janzen and Zenko (2012), American Speech-Language-Hearing Association Practice Policy documents (2006), and the SCERTS Assessment Process (Prizant et al., 2006) for things to consider during the planning phase of an initial evaluation or progress assessment.

Top Ten Tips to Consider before the Assessment

1. Talk with parents, teachers, or other caregivers.

Before beginning the assessment, talk with the child's common caregivers to learn how the child typically communicates in everyday life, how the child typically understands the language around him or her in common contexts, what motivates the child (reinforcers), or situations or materials that might trigger problem behavior or distress.

Be aware that communication levels might be different across various contexts, such as home, school, and out in the community. As discussed previously, there is an incredible range in communication skills within children on the autism spectrum. Does the child use gestures, single words, pictures, an augmentative or alternative communication device, or full spoken sentences? If the child presents with limited verbal communication, it is important to know: how the child indicates their basic needs and wants, any idiosyncratic use of language (e.g., "buh-buh" means water), what strategies help the child understand what others are saying (e.g., gestures, pictures), and if the child answers basic yes and no questions. These answers will be very helpful with structuring the evaluation, so that the child can perform to his or her greatest potential.

2. Review any previous evaluations from medical or educational professionals for insight into the child's individual medical and/or learning profile.

3. Schedule parents, teachers, or other communicative partners to observe and participate in the assessment session.

It is important for familiar caregivers to be a part of the evaluation (Prizant et al., 2006). Many children with ASD may have idiosyncratic communication styles and only those involved with the child will understand their intent (e.g., the child might say "You're a very useful engine!" to communicate that they liked something you did, which is a quote from a popular character on the *Thomas the Tank Engine* television program). As in the example of Cindy above, children with ASD may present with idiosyncratic play skills. It is helpful to get information from caregivers to determine if the child is reenacting a previously experienced event. Familiar caregivers can help the clinician determine if the results of the assessment are representative of the child's typical communication by rating how typical their behavior was. Finally, caregivers can also participate in the evaluation using alternate methods, such as reviewing recordings of the evaluation at a later date and completing checklists and inventories to convey important information about the child's typical communication.

4. Consider the length of testing sessions.

If completing a lengthy evaluation, the examiner may need to schedule multiple, shorter sessions to prevent fatigue and help the child reach his or her potential. Talk with the teachers and/or parents ahead of time to gain information regarding the child's attention skills and how long he or she might be expected to stay on structured tasks.

5. Set up the testing environment to maximize the child's performance.

- Minimize the number and accessibility of items in the environment. For instance, placing too many toys within the child's reach will often lead to the child flitting from one toy to the next. The communicative opportunities will be reduced, because the child has free access to materials and no longer needs a communicative partner.

- Choose materials that encourage interaction. (For example, puzzles and coloring books are most often completed independently and, therefore, do not typically offer many communicative opportunities.)

- If sitting at a table, place the child in the best position to limit auditory, visual distractions. For instance, place the child facing away from reflective surfaces on therapy mirrors, TV monitors, and so forth. Place child away from visual or auditory distractions caused by traffic outside of doorways and windows, near pencil sharpeners, and so forth.

- Provide proper body support for children, particularly those with concomitant motor difficulties, including postural control difficulties. Consider using chairs with backs or sides, and that are at the right height so that children's feet can touch the floor. Children with postural control difficulties may have significant difficulties sitting on the floor in a cross-legged sitting position. Alternative seating, such as sitting on a therapy ball (allows for needed movement), a therapy disk (allows for movement), Rifkin chair, educube, lying on the floor propped up on elbows, and so forth, is often helpful and results in greater attention to task.

6. **Prepare visual supports for use prior to and during the evaluation to explain changes and expectations to the child.**

- Use visual supports at the child's linguistic level. This can be determined or estimated from caregivers' and teachers' descriptions of the child's current communication status or from reviews of previous evaluations. If the child demonstrates low symbolic comprehension (e.g., no use of gestures, signs, pictures, or words to communicate), you will likely need to use nonverbal supports (e.g., all done or a finished box to put materials in that are all done). Language-based visual supports also can vary in complexity: first/then boards, visual schedules with real pictures, visual schedules with line drawings, written schedules with words only, and so forth.

> See Figures 2–6 to 2–9 in Chapter 2 for some samples. Use of visual supports is an excellent evidenced-based strategy, and the reader will find information about visual supports embedded throughout the book.

- Prior to the evaluation, professionals can send an information story to the child to convey what will happen and what to expect during evaluation sessions. The story might contain pictures of the waiting room, the testing room, the examiner(s), and fun materials that the child will interact with, such as toys and books.

> See Appendix A on the accompanying DVD for a sample information story that can be adapted to fit your evaluation setting.

- Make certain that the teacher or parent prepares the child for the change to the existing schedule before test time.

7. Give the child an opportunity to meet you prior to the evaluation.

If providing the evaluation within a school setting, consider visiting the classroom to meet the child in a familiar setting. Professionals working in clinic or educational settings can send an information story to the child with the examiner's picture (see Appendix A on DVD). This often greatly assists the child with transitioning to a new person and setting.

8. Carefully plan the order of assessment activities to alternate easier and more challenging, as well as preferred versus nonpreferred tasks.

Adapt the session schedule to alternate difficult with familiar or easy tasks and breaks. If several difficult or new tasks are presented in a sequence and the failure rate is high, frustration and anxiety will build.

9. Prepare communicative temptations.

When considering evaluation or assessment materials, consider whether or not the activity or material encourages communication with another person. Work to choose activities that allow for natural reasons to communicate, or communicative temptations (Wetherby & Prizant, 1989). The *Communication and Symbolic Behavior Scales* (*CSBS*; Wetherby & Prizant, 1993) contains test items specifically designed to provide opportunities for the child to initiate communication. For instance, one activity involves the use of a balloon. The clinician blows up a balloon and then lets the air out once the child has touched the balloon. The child is given a balloon, which he or she likely cannot blow up alone. Through a sequence described by Wetherby and Prizant (1993), the clinician provides opportunities for the child to initiate a request to have the balloon blown up again. This communicative act might be verbal or nonverbal. Because this activity requires assistance from an adult, it becomes an activity that is shared and provides a communicative temptation.

10. Plan to observe performance in multiple ways.

Using a combination of assessment methods such as parent/teacher reports, observation in natural environments, structured testing, and so forth allows the clinician to see how the child performs when there is little intrusion from the clinician versus significant clinician imposed structure. Particularly when assessing conversational skills, assess the child within multiple situations and environments. For instance, the child could be observed conversing with peers in the lunchroom (nonstructured, group atmosphere), or the child could be assessed having a semistructured conversation about a topic chosen by the examiner in the therapy room (structured, individual setting). Performance across these two situations may be highly variable; children with ASD usually have the most trouble with unstructured, group social settings.

An excellent resource to assist with planning for assessment designed to help with intervention or educational planning is the SCERTS Assessment Process (SAP; Prizant et al., 2006). The SAP utilizes a planning map to help the clinician determine if a balanced assessment has been structured. The clinician documents that multiple observations have been conducted, in multiple locations, at differing times, in at least two natural contexts, in a range of group sizes (individual, small, large groups), over varying activity types. Activities can vary by level of the following aspects: structure, familiarity, difficulty of social requirement (solitary versus social task), preference (preferred versus nonpreferred tasks), language knowledge or use required in the task, activity during learning (passive versus active tasks), and control (child versus adult-led tasks; Prizant et al., 2006).

During the Evaluation

Consideration of the behavioral and cognitive characteristics of individuals with ASD will also help the SLP with problem solving during the assessment. As previously described, children with ASD often have difficulty being flexible with changes to the typical routine, adjusting to a new person or environment, and comprehending language, particularly complex or abstract language. Many assessment tools are utilized in contexts that are more abstract and not in natural contexts the child is accustomed to. There are many strategies that the clinician can employ to help the evaluation process go as smoothly as possible.

- **Allow the child to explore the environment before testing begins.** Remove anything that will likely be a distraction for the child during the assessment. For example, wall decorations that are difficult to redirect the child away from can be removed; reflective surfaces can be covered.

- **Provide a visual schedule and a reinforcement schedule that are individualized to the child.** Giving the child a visual list of tasks to complete helps the child understand how much of the assessment is done and how much is left. This can be a great deterrent of challenging behavior because the concrete nature of a visual schedule is often comforting to the child with ASD. Similarly, a visual reinforcement schedule helps the child maintain motivation by showing the child how he or she will earn rewards during the assessment.

- **Allow the child to be actively involved in monitoring task completion.** Children using visual schedules can assist with crossing out completed items, taking down pictures of completed tasks, and placing pictures in an all done container, or placing actual toys or materials in an all done or finished box. If the child is unable to track the passage of time and is unsure about the end of the session, the individual may appear distracted and disorganized and may exhibit refusal behaviors or try to leave the testing session.

- **Begin assessment with items the child can feel successful with and present a broad range of tasks.** Note that if the child is experiencing delays in language development, the examiner might need to start testing with tasks that are below the child's age level. It also may be beneficial at times to test beyond the standardization criteria to identify more advanced skills. For example, some preschool children with ASD might have knowledge of advanced concepts, such as letters, numbers, or decoding skills despite difficulty with earlier language concepts.

- **Do not repeat directions too many times or too loudly.** Children with ASD have communication difficulties and thus need time to process auditory information. Clinicians should give enough time for the child to process the message and formulate responses, while monitoring for signs that attention has been lost (e.g., looking away, turning away, etc.). Unless the child has a hearing impairment, speaking louder will not assist with comprehension of the message. In fact, the child with ASD may have difficulties with sensory processing and might become overwhelmed by voices that are too loud. Speaking too quickly, loudly, or with frequent repetitions while not allowing for processing time may lead to increased anxiety and subsequent challenging behavior.

- **Consider the age level of the child when choosing materials.** This can be challenging when working with some individuals on the autism spectrum, as there may be a big disparity between developmental level and actual age. For instance, even if a nine-year-old child is nonverbal, the examiner should not present the child with infant or toddler toys during the assessment. The Play Interest Inventory found in *DO-WATCH-LISTEN-SAY* by Quill (2000) discussed in the play section is an excellent resource that can be used to guide observations and parent interviews to help understand the types of materials the child finds interesting and motivating.

- **Be cautious with introduction of highly preferred materials during the assessment.** Remember that by definition, children with ASD often have highly preferred interest areas. Although the examiner wants to utilize materials that are of interest to the child, choose these with caution. Sometimes, the child's special interest area can overpower all other stimuli and make it difficult to shift attention or focus to anything else. It is important to utilize interest areas whenever possible to try and maximize attention and motivation. However, beware of the potential that special interests may have to take over the entire session. Talk with familiar caregivers to help choose the right materials and activities for the assessment.

- **Have materials to prepare quick visual supports.** Materials such as white boards, chalk boards, index cards, paper, and so forth are helpful for visually presenting information as needed. These materials allow the clinician to quickly draw a visual representation for directions, or create a visual cue for increased understanding. For example, drawing a simple T-chart that has first and then columns with pictures and/or words uses the visual processing strengths common in ASD to help ensure understanding and alleviate any anxiety caused by not knowing what is happening next.

See Figure 2–6 for a sample first-then board.

- **Further probe skills from standardized tests to dynamically assess if the child is more successful with alternative prompts, formats, or cues.** Determine the type or level of support needed for the individual to respond correctly. This may mean significant modifications to test formats. Although these modifications might violate standardized test procedures and results, therefore, should not be scored when providing modification, this dynamic assessment will greatly assist with therapy planning, and results can be qualitatively reported.

- **Provide sensorimotor breaks as needed.** Monitor signs of fatigue, negative impacts of sensory elements, or frustration. The child might be observed to appear overwhelmed, such as putting hands over ears or squinting eyes. In contrast, the child might display signs of a low alertness level (e.g., slouching low in chair, lying down on the ground, sucking on fingers, etc.) and need additional sensory stimulation. Providing breaks to go for a walk, get a drink of water, jump on a trampoline, do jumping jacks, have a snack, and so forth often helps the child regain a more optimal level of alertness and be able to sustain attention to the task.

- **End the session on a positive note.** Monitor the child for signs of fatigue and frustration. These signs may be verbal and obvious or might be subtle and/or nonverbal. Be prepared to stop testing if needed and resume on an alternate day. End the session on an item the child feels successful with, and you will be more likely to be able to continue the assessment on another day if needed.

Designing a Comprehensive Social Communication Assessment

What Is Social Communication?

Social communication involves the ability to achieve communicative competence through the child "communicating and playing with others in everyday activities and sharing joy and pleasure in social relationships" (Prizant et al., 2006, p. 3). Communicative competence has been noted in research to be an important predictor of outcomes in adulthood (Garfin & Lord, 1986; McEachin, Smith, & Lovaas, 1993). The SLP provides the expertise to break down the complex process of achieving social communicative competence to determine the best treatment plan to provide remediation. Social communication can be broken down into two foundational components: the capacity for joint attention and for symbol use (Prizant et al., 2006; Wetherby, Prizant, & Schuler, 2000). The following provides more information regarding this framework for breaking down the components of social communication into areas to be assessed during a full communication evaluation.

Joint Attention

Joint attention refers to the capacity to attend to and respond to the social overtures of others through the sharing of attention, emotion, and intentions (Mundy & Stella, 2000; Prizant et al., 2006). Joint attention serves as the foundation for reciprocal communication and should develop across various communication partners and settings (Prizant et al., 2006). Joint attention is a crucial prelinguistic skill for typical language development, as children learn new words in situations when children and a communication partner coordinate their attention toward each other and/or an object (see review of social-pragmatic approach to language acquisition found in Carpenter & Tomasello, 2000). Early language learning stems from the foundational nonlinguistic joint attentional activities (Carpenter, Nagel, & Tomasello, 1998; Carpenter & Tomasello, 2000). In young children, this often happens in everyday routines, such as during diaper changes, mealtime, bathing routines, and so forth. As typically developing children pass beyond their first birthdays, they continue to learn cognitive and linguistic information through joint attention directed toward adults and imitation of what they observe (Carpenter & Tomasello, 2000).

Unique Characteristics of Joint Attention in Children with ASD

Children with ASD present with a basic difficulty with "following into and directing others' attention and interest to objects in their shared world" (Carpenter & Tomasello, 2000, p. 42). This significant difficulty with establishing joint attention leads to decreased language learning and is a powerful indicator of the presence of ASD in young children (Carpenter & Tomasello, 2000; Mundy & Stella, 2000). As a matter of fact, decreased joint attention "appears to be a hallmark of autism and is not characteristic of children with developmental language disorders or mental retardation" (Wetherby et al., 2000, p. 110). Examples of joint attention difficulties that may be observed in children with ASD (Carpenter & Tomasello, 2000; Gutstein & Sheely, 2002; Mundy & Stella, 2000; Prizant et al., 2006):

- Difficulty orienting to speech sounds in infancy
- Reduced referential looking: Alternating eye gaze back and forth between objects of focus and adult's faces
- Decreased pointing and showing
- Difficulty with following others' attentional focus, such as looking toward a point or looking toward where an individual is looking
- Reduced social referencing
- Decreased use of gestures paired with attentional focus at the communication partner the gesture is intended for
- In verbal children, may observe difficulty following and using eye gaze during conversational exchanges. Child may have difficulty with turn-taking, particularly with participating in conversations with more than one person where speaker-listener roles change frequently.

Symbol Use: The Content and Form of Language

Symbol use refers to a foundational concept that gives rise to both language and play development, specifically the child's comprehension of shared meanings (Bates, 1979;

Prizant et al., 2006; Wetherby & Prizant, 1993). This includes: comprehension or use of nonverbal forms of communication (e.g., gestures, vocalizations, facial expressions, etc.), comprehension or use of words and combinations of words, the development of object use and play development, and comprehension or use of social conventions used in reciprocal communication (Prizant et al., 2006). This is the aspect most typically assessed by SLPs and the component of social communication that SLPs are usually given the most training in. To equate to known schemas, symbol use refers to the *content* and the *form* in the model by Bloom and Lahey (1978), whereas joint attention serves as the foundation of *use*. Similarly, symbol use refers to the semantics, syntax, and morphology usage. Figure 3–1 illustrates the connections between cognitive components, linguistic aspects, and external influences.

Unique Characteristics of Symbolic Language in Children with ASD

Children with ASD often have difficulty with developing "conventional and symbolic aspects of communication" (Wetherby et al., 2000, p. 113). This includes a reduction in gestural use (Wetherby et al., 2000). Children with ASD are observed to have an extended period of use of presymbolic gestures, such as using the caregiver's hand as a tool by placing the person's hand on a desired item (Prizant et al., 2006). It is also important to note that some children with ASD, who are at a presymbolic level, may also be observed

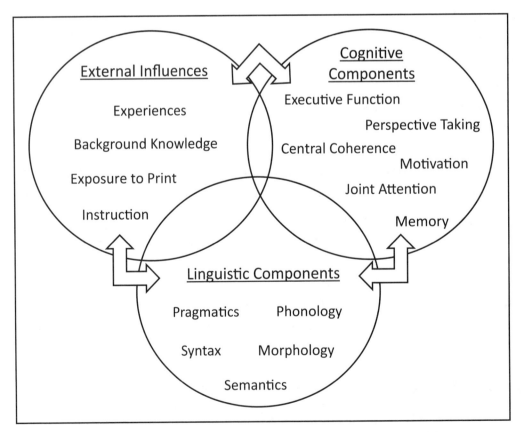

Figure 3–1. Relationships between cognitive, linguistic, and external factors.

to use problem behaviors as a means to communicate (Fox, Dunlap, & Buschbacher, 2000; Prizant et al., 2006).

The cognitive and learning characteristics of individuals with ASD help explain the way they acquire language. Research demonstrates that individuals with ASD are more likely to be gestalt processors (rote memory for larger chunks of language with or without comprehension), rather than analytic processors (acquire language through a hierarchy, moving up in linguistic complexity from single words, two word utterances, etc.; Prizant et al., 2006). Relatedly, children with ASD are often observed to exactly reenact events or parts of events to communicate, often to request. As children with ASD learn to increase their symbolic understanding, they may need to go through an extended period of reenactments, including use of echolalia (Prizant et al., 2006). Echolalia is frequently seen in children with ASD as they are noted to sometimes immediately repeat what was just said (immediate echolalia) or later repeat multiword utterances heard previously (delayed echolalia; Prizant et al., 2006). These repetitions of whole chunks of language are consistent with the processing style of children with ASD (i.e., gestalt processing). Echolalia actually can serve many communicative functions, including requesting, protesting, affirming, calling, labeling, providing information, or giving a directive (Prizant & Rydell, 1984). Echolalia might help the child by serving as: (1) a learning strategy for the child with ASD similar to imitation noted in typically developing children, (2) rehearsal to assist with memory and comprehension, or (3) self-talk to assist the child with completing a task (Prizant & Rydell, 1984; Prizant et al., 2006).

Because children with ASD may have more difficulty breaking language down analytically, the clinician should be careful to assess the full range of language skills when assessing communication in verbal children with ASD. For instance, single-word vocabulary skills may be significantly higher than comprehension or expression of multiword utterances (e.g., sentences, discourse; Klin et al., 2005). There is a large variation in the types of oral language skills seen in children with ASD, and errors may or may not be seen in structural language skills (phonology, semantics, syntax; Tager-Flusberg, Paul, & Lord, 2005).

> See Case Study B–1 on the accompanying DVD for a video example of a child with conversational language difficulties without structural language difficulties.

The SLP will need to assess all aspects of language (semantics, syntax, phonology, morphology, and pragmatics) within a comprehensive communication evaluation. In summary, types of communication behaviors that are often seen in children with ASD (Paul, 2005; Prizant et al., 2006):

- Echolalia (immediate, delayed, mitigated)
- Misuse of pronouns or pronoun reversals

- Idiosyncratic language
- Verbal routines
- Decreased pragmatic language
- Decreased responsiveness to speech.

Components of a Social Communication Assessment

Specific areas to assess within a social communication assessment differ depending on the level of verbal communication: preverbal, emerging verbal, or fluently verbal. This is consistent with several models designed to assist with intervention play development. The SCERTS model describes these broad developmental stages as beginning with the social partner, where the child learns to intentionally communicate using gestures or vocalizations (Prizant et al., 2006). The next stage of emerging verbal children is labeled the language partner stage within the SCERTS model, as this stage marks the time when first words and word combinations begin (Prizant et al., 2006). The final broad phase of social communication development described within the SCERTS model is the conversational partner stage, which is marked by children's expanding sentence constructions and emergence of conversational discourse (Prizant et al., 2006). Another example of a framework for the progression of communication is described by MacDonald (2004) as a continuum containing the following five overlapping stages: interaction, nonverbal communication, social language, conversation, and civil behavior. Understanding where the child falls in the general progression of social communication will assist the evaluator with designing a comprehensive evaluation. The following lists identify areas to consider when designing a comprehensive social communication assessment battery for children across varying levels of linguistic development (see Klin et al., 2005; National Research Council, 2001; Paul, 2005).

Preverbal:
- Language comprehension
- Language expression (including possible use of signs, AAC to communicate)
- Communicative acts
- Joint attention
- Phonemic repertoire for any vocalizations
- Oral structures and function
- Play skills: Symbolic and social levels
- Voice and resonance during any vocalizations
- Refer to audiology for complete hearing evaluation.

Emerging Verbal:
- Language skills across all areas: Semantics, syntax, morphology, phonology, and pragmatics

- Communicative acts
- Social reciprocity or joint attention
- Play skills: Symbolic and social
- Emergent literacy
- Speech sound development
- Oral structures and function
- Voice, resonance, and fluency
- Prosody
- Hearing (screen and/or refer to audiology for a complete hearing evaluation).

Fluently Verbal:

- Language skills across all areas: Semantics, syntax, morphology, phonology, and pragmatics
  - Assess in both oral and written domains
  - Be sure to assess language along the range of length and complexity, including up to conversational discourse
  - Nonliteral language development (e.g., metaphors, sarcasm, humor)
  - Comprehension of words with multiple meanings
  - Language flexibility
- Social reciprocity or joint attention
- Perspective taking skills or theory of mind
- Social skills
- Play skills and/or peer relationships
- Literacy development:
  - word recognition and decoding
  - spelling
  - reading comprehension (explicit and implicit information)
  - written expression
- Speech sound development
- Oral structures and function if speech sound disorder is present (SSD)
- Prosody
- Voice, resonance, and fluency
- Hearing screening; Refer to audiology for a complete audiological evaluation if reliability is compromised.

A social communication assessment for a child diagnosed with or suspected of having ASD includes many of the standard areas found in any communication evaluation. There are particular areas, included in the lists above, which are suspect when evaluating children with autism. Many of these areas are due to the core criteria associated with a diagnosis of ASD (e.g., social skills difficulties are prerequisite to a diagnosis), whereas other areas are not prerequisite, but are often observed in children with ASD (e.g., motor speech difficulties). Areas of specific importance to a social communication evaluation with a child suspected of having or being diagnosed with ASD are discussed in further detail below.

Assessing the Communicative Act

A helpful framework for assessing communication is in terms of communicative acts and functions. According to Shumway and Wetherby (2009), a communicative act is "an interactive behavior that consists of a gesture, vocalization, or verbalization that is directed toward another person and that serves a communicative function" (p. 1144). Communicative functions are the reasons why we communicate and can be divided into three main categories: behavior regulation, social interaction, and joint attention (Bruner, 1981). The first communicative functions to appear fall in the behavior regulation category, meaning the child is communicating to alter the behavior of another person to fulfill a need. In this early developmental stage, a child uses any communicative act to request something from another person or to protest something another person is doing to get them to stop (Bruner, 1981; Shumway & Wetherby, 2009; Wetherby & Prizant, 2002). Social interaction is the next category of communicative functions that develops when a child tries to attract or maintain another person's attention. Finally, communicative acts conveyed to achieve joint attention involve directing another person's attention to an object, event, or topic in the form of commenting or requesting more information (Bruner, 1981; Shumway & Wetherby, 2009; Wetherby & Prizant, 2002). The progression of communicative function categories start with meeting a child's personal needs and moves toward communicating to share and gain social or emotional reciprocity. This progression is important to understand, as children with ASD tend to use language for primarily instrumental functions, or to regulate the behaviors of others (Mundy & Stella, 2000; Prizant et al., 2006). This includes primary functions to get others to do something (request) or to get someone to stop doing something (protest) (Wetherby et al., 2000).

Viewing children's communication from the perspective of communicative acts is especially helpful when assessing the language use of children with ASD. Many standardized language measures commonly used by the SLP focus on one aspect of communication, particularly the form of language, with less focus being given to the functions of the communication (Wetherby & Prizant, 1993). To truly gain insight into the communication skills of children with ASD, it is important to look beyond syntax, semantics, and morphology. The clinician also needs to look at why and when the child communicates. For instance, does the child solely communicate to get his or her needs and wants met (i.e., instrumental functions only)? Does the child communicate with the purpose of socially interacting? Does the child initiate communicative interactions? These are important questions to answer when designing a comprehensive intervention plan.

Clinicians can utilize conversational language sampling to gain insight into children's spontaneous social communication. There are several checklists the clinician can utilize to assist with structuring the analysis of the sample, including Prutting and Kirchner's

(1987) Pragmatic Protocol and the Systematic Observation of Communicative Interaction (Damico, Oller, & Tetnowski, 1999). The *Communication and Symbolic Behavior Scales* (*CSBS*; Wetherby & Prizant, 1993) is a helpful standardized tool for the clinician to structure and analyze the assessment of communicative acts. The measure provides a structured format to elicit social communication and play using communicative temptations, or activities specifically designed to encourage the child's conversation and interaction.

Play Assessment

In typical development, play development parallels language achievements (Bates, O'Connell, & Shore, 1987; McCune-Nicolich & Carroll, 1981). This makes sense when one considers that both play and language emerge as symbolic understanding develops in children. Both play and language are symbol systems that result from the understanding that one thing can stand for and represent something else (Bates, 1979). These skills are both also acquired within a social context of sharing attention on objects (Prizant et al., 2006). For example, as children develop first words, they also typically develop single action play schemes; as they begin combining words, they also begin combining actions in play schemes. Play is also an important way that children develop understanding of social conventions as they act out routines and roles they experience in their environment and to develop interpersonal skills with one another (Beyer & Gammeltoft, 1998). Therefore, the SLP plays an important role in assessing the components of play and helping to make connections between the child's play and social communication development. This assessment will assist the SLP with the design of individualized treatment plans that include goals targeting the child's underlying difficulty with play development.

Play skills can be viewed from two perspectives; both in the level of symbolism demonstrated and how the play involves others socially (Quill, 2000; Wolfberg, 2009). Therefore, it is important to look at both dimensions of play when assessing this area. Play develops along a social continuum, with the child moving from the ability to play independently to being a member of coordinated group play (Wolfberg, 2009). The development of symbolic understanding rises from social attention and imitation; children gradually move from immediately imitating the actions of others to imitating actions and action sequences at later times (Prizant et al., 2006). This imitation assists with learning about the functional uses of common objects in the child's environment, which gives rise to functional symbolic play. As children with ASD have difficulties with joint attention, they often present with decreased spontaneous imitation skills due to decreased sharing of attention and experiences (Prizant et al., 2006). According to the DSM-IV-TR children with ASD might demonstrate "lack of varied, spontaneous make-believe play or social imitative play appropriate to developmental level" (American Psychiatric Association, 2000, p. 75). Because of these difficulties with developing play skills, children with ASD often also have difficulties participating in the surrounding peer culture and with developing relationships with peers (Wolfberg, 1999). For more in-depth information regarding play development and assessment, see *Peer Play and the Autism Spectrum: The Art of Guiding Children's Socialization and Imagination* (Wolfberg, 2003).

Symbolic Play

Typical symbolic play development begins with the young child exploring his or her environment using the senses, for example by mouthing, grasping, dropping, and so forth (Wolfberg, 2003). The classic example is the young child mouthing toys during play. Symbolism within play progresses as children begin to manipulate objects in their environment. This includes expanding manipulation play to learn cause-effect relationships with objects and combining objects within sensorimotor play (e.g., filling and dumping, banging objects together, etc.; Wolfberg, 2003). The child then learns functional relationships of objects and uses this knowledge within play. Functional play begins with simple actions and progresses to more complex schemas (Wolfberg, 2003). For instance, the child may begin to play with a toy phone as an actual telephone and pretend to talk into it. Finally, symbolic-pretend play is seen when children begin to represent events they have experienced within their play (e.g., pretending to pour tea into cups despite no liquid being present). The complexity of symbolic-pretend play progresses in the preschool years as children incorporate imaginary objects, themes, and take on multiple roles within play schemas. For instance, the child may pretend that he and his teddy bear are astronauts about to take off in their spaceship to go on a mission to the moon.

In contrast, children with ASD have difficulty developing symbolic play skills in a typical manner and sequence (Wolfberg, 1999). Manipulation play is frequently seen for extended periods of time and may be observed to be more repetitive and restricted than typically developing peers in this phase (Wolfberg, 2003). Children with ASD may have inflexible play schemas and may play in stereotypical ways (Beyer & Gammeltoft, 1998). The sensory processing differences associated with many children on the autism spectrum may lead to increased focus on sensorimotor exploration of their environment. Their exploration may also become ritualized and stereotypic routines may be observed (Wolfberg, 2003). For instance, during an observational assessment on a three-year-old child within the preschool setting, the authors observed the child wandering around the playground tipping all wheeled toys (bikes, play cars, wagons, etc.) upside down and watching the wheels slowly turn around before moving to the next wheeled item. Functional and pretend play are often decreased or absent in the play routines of children with ASD. Additionally, children with ASD are often noted to have differences in how functional play is conducted, including less diverse play scripts (Wolfberg, 2003). When symbolic-pretend play is observed, it may be surrounding specific areas of interest and may contain scripts from recent events, television programs, and so forth (Beyer & Gammeltoft, 1998).

There are many different types of play activities and materials. These differing types of play can yield qualitatively different results during observational assessments. For instance, observation of bike riding will often lead to observation of solitary play and may not yield needed information regarding social play skills. It is also important to be aware of the types of play because children with ASD may have differing abilities across types of activities. For instance, children with ASD frequently demonstrate similar or near similar to typically developing children on constructive play activities because visual-spatial problem solving is often an area of strength (Prizant et al., 2006). In contrast, performance within other types of play are usually significantly decreased. One framework for assessment of play types is presented by Quill (2000) in her Play Interest Survey found in the *DO-WATCH-LISTEN-SAY* text. This checklist can be given to parents and teachers to assist the examiner with gleaning information about skills demonstrated outside of a clinical context. Within Quill's framework, she identifies the following types of play:

- Exploratory play (e.g., sandbox, bubbles)
- Physical play (e.g., bike riding, swinging)
- Manipulatives (e.g., use of shape sorters, Mr. Potato Head)
- Constructive play (e.g., use of Legos, K'Nex)
- Art (e.g., painting, coloring)
- Literacy (e.g., playing with ABC toys such as magnetic letters, talking books)
- Sociodramatic play (e.g., playing with barn and animals, makeup, and costumes)
- Games (e.g., Uno, Candy Land)
- Music (e.g., musical toys or instruments)
- Social games (e.g., peek-a-boo, hide and seek)

Symbolic play skills can be assessed through careful observational assessment. The clinician should note the type of context and level of structure when observing play and try to observe multiple contexts, levels of structure, and types of play activities and materials. For instance, the child in a preschool classroom who is given free reign to choose any toys within the room might be observed to only choose solitary tasks such as the computer or reading books by him or herself. The same child might present very differently when the teacher on another day structures the children to rotate through several organized centers and, thus, the child is forced to demonstrate play skills outside of his or her preferred interest areas. As discussed previously, the SCERTS model's *SAP map* is a helpful tool for clinicians to plan a balanced assessment (see Prizant et al., 2006). Use of observational checklists are helpful for guiding one's observation, such as the framework found in *Peer Play and the Autism Spectrum* (Wolfberg, 2003) and the Social Play Task Analysis found in *DO-WATCH-LISTEN-SAY* (Quill, 2000). Keep in mind that observations of play skills of children with ASD might be very different in a one-on-one clinical setting with an adult versus a group setting with peers. Those clinicians in an educational setting should observe play skills within natural play opportunities in the child's day. For those clinicians in center- or clinic-based environments, parent and teacher interviews can assist with comparing skills observed in the therapy room with skills with peers in natural contexts. For instance, the play portion of the *Assessment of Social and Communication Skills for Children with Autism* can be used to structure the interview with a caregiver (Quill, 2000). When assessing the child's symbolic play skills, the clinician should seek the answer to the question, "How does the child play with toys?" Figure 3–2 illustrates the progression of play development for typically developing children.

Symbolic Dimension of Play
Observational Framework

- **Sensorimotor Play**: Also called Exploratory/ Manipulation play. Involves sensory experiences with objects, such as sucking, throwing, spinning, rolling, and so forth. Typically developed within the first six to eight months of age.
- **Organizing Play**: Child begins ordering objects in the environment, although this organization may not be based on a specific rationale for categorization. Children can be seen stacking items, putting them inside one another, and so forth. Typically developed from six to nine months of age.
- **Functional Play**: Play involves appropriate use of an object in play. For example, rolling a car, placing a cup on a saucer. This play rises from social imitation in the typically developing child. Typically observed to develop from 9 to 12 months.
- **Symbolic—Pretend Play**: Child can pretend one object is another, imagine pretend aspects of play— pretend a banana is a telephone; pretend a cup has tea in it. Routine scripts emerge first about familiar themes. Sociodramatic play emerges. Typically noted to emerge from around 18 months and beyond.

Figure 3–2. A framework of the developmental progression of symbolic play (Adapted from Wolfberg, 2003; Quill, 2000; Beyer & Gammeltoft, 1998).

Social Play

Play also develops along a social continuum, with the child moving from the ability to play independently to being able to be a member of coordinated group play (Wolfberg, 2009). Play serves as the context for typically developing children to expand their understanding about social dynamics and to develop relationships and friendships (Wolfberg, 1999, 2009). Although different sources may use varying terminology for the *phases* of typical social play development, the progression of skills remains consistent. Children initially learn to engage socially with caregivers through attending to their actions, such as facial expressions and vocalizations, imitating what they see. This social imitation is the foundation for developing the social aspects of play. Wolfberg (2003) describes that children next become *onlookers* in which they watch peers playing, learning about peer culture and play routines prior to engaging in more coordinated play with them. Typically developing children then can be observed *parallel* playing, whereby they play in the vicinity of peers and with similar materials. Eventually, the children can play with a *common focus* and begin to interact with peers during play routines. Finally, typically developing children will eventually learn to have shared goals within play, such as playing a game together, acting out a common story or event, or constructing something together (e.g., collaboratively building a sandcastle, making an art project, etc.). Children with ASD have difficulty with joint attention and social imitation, which decreases their availability to learn higher level social play skills (i.e., playing with a common focus and playing collaboratively which both require well-developed joint attention and imitation skills to achieve). Although social play is overall an area of difficulty for children with ASD, their specific skills within this area often present very differently from individual to individual. Children with ASD may have difficulty responding to peers' attempts to play, initiating play with peers, and/or with playing appropriately with peers (Quill, 2000; Wolfberg, 2003). Again, these difficulties are reflective of their underlying deficits in the area of joint attention and mirror social communication difficulties. For instance, a child who has difficulty maintaining a topic within a play routine being acted out by a peer (e.g., continually tries to turn a game of house into dinosaurs as the play routine progresses) will usually also demonstrate difficulty with topic maintenance during communication. When assessing the child's social play skills, the clinician should seek the answer to the question, "How does the child play with people?" Children's social play development is best assessed using an observational assessment within a natural context for the child (e.g., preschool, play group). Again, observational checklists and frameworks greatly assist the examiner as discussed in the symbolic play section. Figure 3–3 lists a general progression of skills along the social play continuum discussed by Wolfberg (2003) within her framework for assessing children prior to participating in integrated play groups.

Whereas the symbolic and social aspects of play tend to develop in tandem within typically developing children, the clinician should be prepared for variations to this when assessing children with ASD. Although these skills may develop in parallel, the clinician may also see discrepancies such as those demonstrated in the profile below for Adam (Figure 3–4). Adam's symbolic play development reveals he is developing at the highest level of symbolic play, the pretend play level. However, the social aspect of play remains at the Onlooker level, demonstrating that he continues to have difficulties with underlying joint attention and social interaction skills. Adam's verbal communication skills mirror this; he frequently produces sentences appropriate for his age to comment

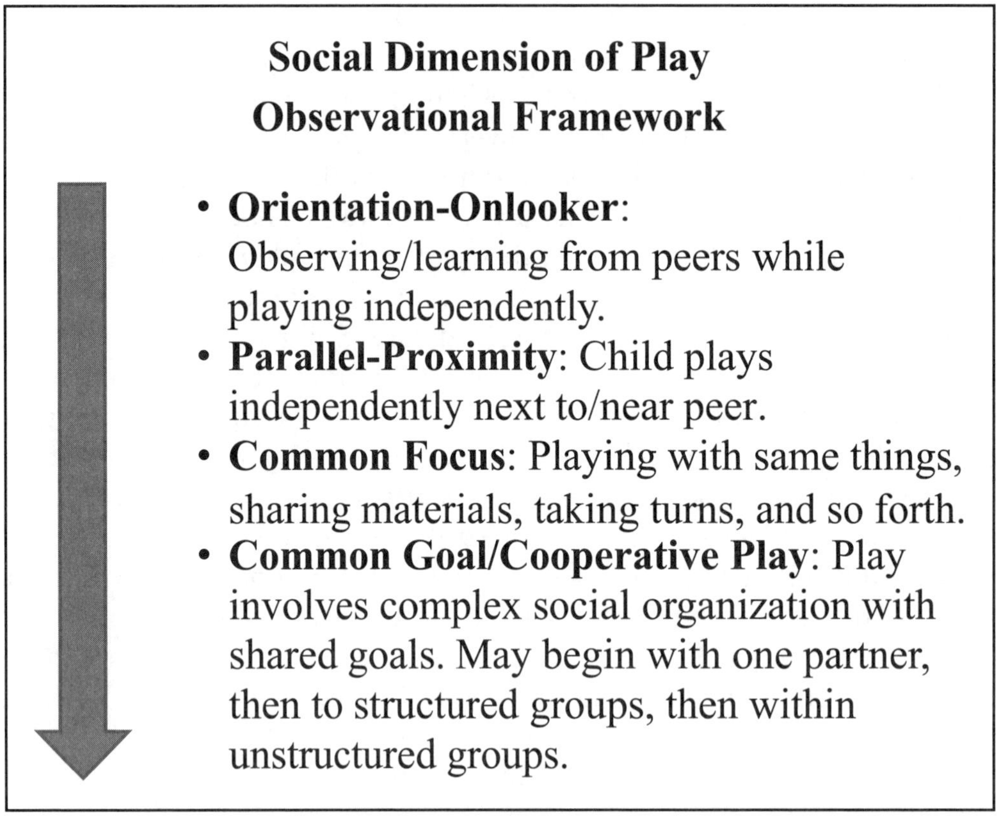

Social Dimension of Play
Observational Framework

- **Orientation-Onlooker**: Observing/learning from peers while playing independently.
- **Parallel-Proximity**: Child plays independently next to/near peer.
- **Common Focus**: Playing with same things, sharing materials, taking turns, and so forth.
- **Common Goal/Cooperative Play**: Play involves complex social organization with shared goals. May begin with one partner, then to structured groups, then within unstructured groups.

Figure 3–3. A framework of the developmental progression of the social dimension of play (Adapted from Wolfberg, 2003; Quill, 2000).

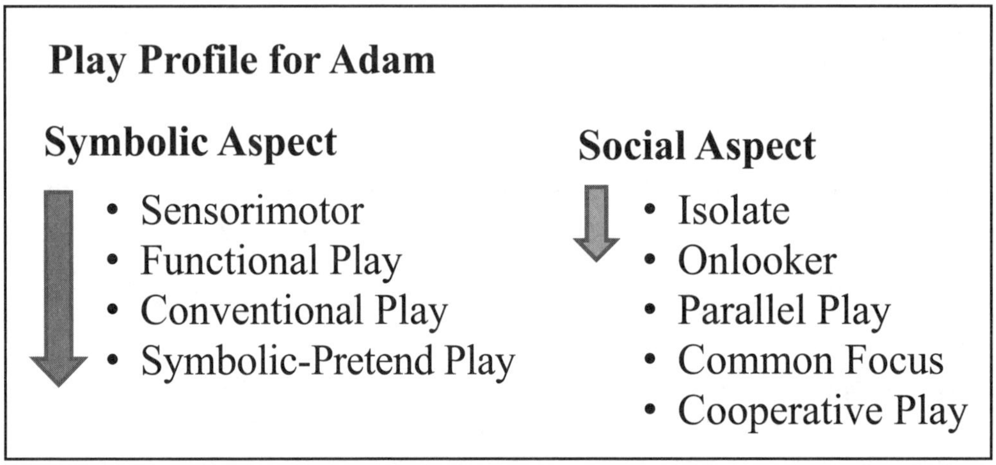

Play Profile for Adam

Symbolic Aspect

- Sensorimotor
- Functional Play
- Conventional Play
- Symbolic-Pretend Play

Social Aspect

- Isolate
- Onlooker
- Parallel Play
- Common Focus
- Cooperative Play

Figure 3–4. A profile of play development across both symbolic and social dimensions.

about things and events in his environment and has been observed to have a sizable vocabulary. However, Adam does not yet have back and forth conversations where he consistently responds, takes conversational turns, maintains topic, and so forth. He does verbally comment on things in his environment; however, his comments are not usually directed toward others for a social purpose.

Assessment of Speech

When assessing the speech of children with ASD, there are some unique considerations to be made. First, children with ASD have been noted to have increased rates of speech sound disorders (SSDs), particularly distortions in verbal children (Shriberg, Paul, Black, & Van Santen, 2011). Although a SSD is not a part of the core criteria for ASD and many children with ASD in fact do not have any difficulties with speech sound development, the SLP should be prepared to assess this area. Additionally, research has shown an increase in difficulty with motor skill development, including apraxia, in those diagnosed with ASD (Ming, Brimacombe, & Wagner, 2007). Therefore, the SLP should be on the lookout for signs and symptoms of childhood apraxia of speech (CAS) or dysarthria when the child presents with a speech sound disorder. CAS in particular has been theorized to be a possible reason for some children with ASD remaining nonverbal; however, this continues to be debated (Shriberg et al., 2011). Please see the American Speech-Language-Hearing Association's position statement on CAS, including the definition and key criteria (American Speech-Language-Hearing Association, 2007).

Relatedly, children with ASD have commonly been noted to have difficulty with the production of prosody, or the musical/suprasegmental aspects of speech including pitch, duration, and intensity (Grossman, Bemis, Skwerer, & Tager-Flusberg, 2010; Paul, 2005). A review by Shriberg, Paul, McSweeny, Klin, Cohen, and Volkmar (2001) summarized aspects of prosody in the following areas: grammatical prosody (signals syntactic information), pragmatic prosody (conveys social information), and affective prosody (communicates the speaker's emotions, use of varying registers, and the personal speech style of the speaker). The following aspects of prosody have been noted to be difficult in a significant number of children with ASD (Shriberg et al., 2011; Shriberg et al., 2001):

- Atypical use of stress
- Disfluency, characterized by inappropriate or nonfluent phrasing (increased repetitions and revisions)
- Increased intensity/loudness
- Use of higher pitch
- Increased nasality.

Prosody has historically been an area commonly reported to be atypical in individuals with ASD. The difficulties previously described may have a negative impact on the child's success with communication. In terms of assessment, Paul (2005) recommended clinical evaluation of prosody during speech/language sampling. She recommended the clinician evaluate the following areas in particular: stress, volume, fluency, intonation, and nasality. A descriptive scale can be used, such as "appropriate, inappropriate, no opportunity to observe" (Paul, 2005, p. 814).

Written Communication: An Important Piece of the Communication Assessment

Written communication is an important area to assess for all children with communication disorders, including children with ASD. Written language development is truly part of the continuum of language development that continues into the adult years (Westby, 2002). According to the American Speech-Language-Hearing Association's *Professional Issues Statement on Roles and Responsibilities of Speech-Language Pathologists in the Schools,* "current research supports the interrelationships across the language processes of listening, speaking, reading, and writing" (American Speech-Language-Hearing Association, 2010). Because of these interrelationships, research has shown that children with language disorders are at greater risk for written language disorders, with oral language difficulties being sometimes a cause and sometimes a consequence of literacy difficulties (Catts, Fey, Zhang, & Tomblin, 1999; Catts & Kamhi, 1999; Snow, Burns, & Griffin, 1998). In fact, the definition of a language disorder put forth in an official statement by the American Speech-Language-Hearing Association (1993) includes both written and spoken aspects of language, specifically: "a language disorder is impaired comprehension and/or use of spoken, written and/or other symbol systems." Because children with ASD by definition demonstrate some type of difficulty in the area of communication, difficulty with literacy development is expected, although the types of difficulty with literacy may vary greatly (Nation, Clarke, Wright, & Williams, 2006). The SLP can draw on familiar schemas related to spoken language development to help identify where breakdowns occur and how deficits in underlying linguistic knowledge can negatively affect both spoken and written language. See Table 3–1 for a summary of the relationship between spoken and written language.

Research has shown that children with ASD display a wide range of literacy skills, and there is not one profile of literacy development associated with a diagnosis of ASD (Jones et al., 2009; Norbury & Nation, 2011). Children with ASD can have difficulty with any one or more aspects of literacy (word recognition, decoding, spelling, reading comprehension, writing; Estes, Rivera, Bryan, Cali, & Dawson, 2011; Jones et al., 2009; Norbury &

Table 3–1. Relationships Between Linguistic Components and Written Language

Linguistic Components		Related Areas of Literacy
CONTENT	• Semantics • Morphology	• Word Recognition • Reading Comprehension
FORM	• Phonology • Syntax	• Decoding • Encoding • Writing: Sentence Construction
USE	• Pragmatics	• Written Expression • Reading Comprehension

Nation, 2011). It is important to note that there are some children with ASD who acquire literacy despite significant oral language delay, even those who are nonverbal (Norbury & Nation, 2011). In fact, many children with ASD have strengths in some aspect of written language development (Estes et al., 2011). This was demonstrated in the case example of Cindy above.

There is a subset of children with ASD that may present with what has been termed hyperlexia, or superior word recognition skills despite cognitive linguistic difficulties that also lead to poor reading comprehension (Grigorenko, Klin, & Volkmar, 2003). There is some debate regarding all features associated with hyperlexia (e.g., some suggest an unusual preoccupation with reading is part of the core features), with how common the phenomenon is in the population with ASD, if hyperlexia extends beyond the diagnostic category of ASD to other developmental disorders, and whether or not the phenomenon exists outside of the population with developmental delays (Grigorenko et al., 2003). Regardless of the terminology used, the SLP should use a comprehensive assessment of all aspects of literacy to determine the best course of action in intervention. This assessment will be the most valuable tool for planning balanced intervention rather than a diagnostic label (e.g., hyperlexia).

When evaluating the literacy development of a child with ASD, the SLP must determine the spoken and written communication profile for that individual child with ASD. The clinician is looking to figure out: (1) which aspects of literacy development are not developing at chronological or expected grade level (i.e., reading, spelling, writing), (2) which processes are difficult for the child and leading to delayed reading, spelling, and writing, and (3) how do the difficulties with written language compare with deficits in related cognitive and linguistic skills. Questions that should be answered within the assessment might include: Does the child have difficulty with reading or spelling the words? Does the child read the words fluently but have difficulty reading for meaning? Does the child have trouble with both reading the words and also reading for meaning? Does the child have trouble with just spelling or spelling as well as composing written language? A comprehensive evaluation of written communication skills includes the following areas, as applicable for age and developmental level:

- Oral language skills: Single words up to discourse level; all aspects including content/form/use; semantics, syntax, phonology, morphology, pragmatics
- Emergent literacy skills: Print awareness, phonological awareness, letter knowledge
- Phonemic awareness
- Single-word reading and spelling skills
- Connected reading skills (reading accuracy, fluency)
- Reading comprehension
- Writing composition.

Test results can be looked at several ways. First, an overall profile can be determined regarding which literacy skills are areas of strengths and concern. Second, clinicians can analyze for profiles within the test to determine the reasons for delays. For instance, the clinician might note that during the reading comprehension assessment using the QRI-5, the child answered all questions that were related to recalling specific details (explicit questions) and typically missed questions requiring further analysis of implicit information (e.g., inferencing, prediction, etc.). Third, the SLP can analyze results across tests, such as comparing specific oral language skills with written language skills, to better understand reasons for breakdowns occurring in literacy. For instance, a child might present with excellent single-word vocabulary, yet progressive difficulty with comprehension of language as it increases in length to complex sentences and stories (discourse). This same child might similarly have a strength in the area of word recognition, which is correlated with vocabulary skills, but significant difficulty on measures of reading comprehension. Another example could include comparison of specific skills, such as observing that a child has difficulty with identifying words that are similar on the Word Classes subtests of the CELF-4 and likewise noting that the child consistently missed questions regarding main idea during the reading comprehension assessment using the GORT-5. Understanding how concepts can be similar or related is a precursor to understanding how multiple key details in stories are similar (i.e., what the main idea is of the most important details in a story). These connections are especially helpful during assessment for planning intervention and educational plans and serve as a map for how to integrate oral and written language targets in therapy.

> See Chapter 6 for in-depth information regarding written communication of children with ASD, including analysis of findings to set goals.

Diagnosis and Coding

As previously discussed, early identification of children with ASD is paramount to provide early intervention (National Research Council, 2001). Evaluations for diagnosis of ASD should be conducted by clinicians who have a knowledge base in the area of ASD (Filipek et al., 1999; National Research Council, 2001). According to the American Speech-Language-Hearing Association (2006) practice policy documents for SLPs working with children suspected of having ASD, "ideally the diagnostic role of the SLP would be as a key member of an interdisciplinary team with the appropriate individual and collective expertise in ASD." The independent SLP with no additional training in the area of ASD should refer the child to a team of professionals who can provide the comprehensive evaluation to determine if an ASD is present. Under the current DSM-5 (American Psychiatric Association, 2013) SLPs can now specify that the nature of a child's language disorder includes difficulty with social communication rather than solely a more generalized language learning disorder. More specific, SLPs can give the diagnosis of Social (Pragmatic) Communication Disorder, which is under the broader diagnostic category of

Communication Disorder. This code will help communicate that a pragmatic language disorder specifically is present and assist the interdisciplinary team that you refer the child to by documenting the presence of one of the two main components of the diagnosis of ASD (i.e., social communication).

Referrals

As stated in the section above, it is imperative that a team of professionals collaborate when working with children with ASD. This includes "appropriate referrals to rule out other conditions and facilitate access to comprehensive services" (American Speech-Language-Hearing Association, 2006). It is important that the SLP understand the nature of ASD and the related conditions so that proper referrals can be made. The SLP working with a child suspected of having ASD should ensure that a *medical team* is involved in the early stages of diagnosis. Initial medical evaluations for children being assessed for a possible ASD should rule out other possible causes for symptomatology, including: vision status, hearing status, genetic conditions (e.g., fragile X syndrome) or metabolic disorders (American Speech-Language-Hearing Association, 2006; Filipek et al., 1999; National Research Council, 2001). Whereas SLPs conduct hearing screenings within their scope of practice, the clinician should be prepared to refer to a *pediatric audiologist* if behavioral or developmental difficulties make it difficult to conduct the screening. Additionally, a higher incidence of seizure disorders has been noted in children with ASD, and the child should be referred for a *neurological evaluation* if symptoms are noted, such as staring spells (National Research Council, 2001). Motor disorders commonly cooccur in children with ASD, so the SLP may need to refer to an *occupational or physical therapist* to assess gross and/or fine motor skills (National Research Council, 2001). According to a review by Ming et al. (2007), these motor difficulties might include delayed gross and/or fine motor development, hypotonia, apraxia, decreased postural control, toe-walking, or overall incoordination.

Finally, children with ASD are at significantly increased risk for the presence of *anxiety and depression* (Kim, Szatmari, Bryson, Streiner, & Wilson, 2000; Van Steensel, Bögels, & Perrin, 2011). In a recent meta-analysis by Van Steensel et al. (2011), close to 40% of the individuals with ASD across the studies analyzed were noted to present with some type of anxiety disorder. It is important for SLPs to be aware that children with ASD may have related areas of difficulty. As discussed previously, SLPs may be among the first professionals consulted when a child is suspected of having ASD and should be able to refer children to get the help they need.

Resources: Speech Language Assessments Helpful for Use with ASD

The following is a list of resources that may be helpful to the clinician designing a comprehensive communication evaluation or ongoing assessment for children with ASD. The clinician should use clinical judgment when choosing which of the following materials might be appropriate for individual children with ASD. The discussion within this chapter should provide the clinician with guidance regarding the types of measures that will be most effective. This list is by no means exhaustive, rather a list of resources that are frequently utilized within assessments focused on social communication in particular.

Language

- *Clinical Evaluation of Language Fundamentals-Fourth Edition* (*CELF-4*; Semel, Wiig, & Secord, 2003).
  - Note: The *Clinical Evaluation of Language Fundamental-Fifth Edition* (*CELF-5*) is due out in fall of 2013 (Semel, Wiig, & Secord, in press).
- *Clinical Evaluation of Language Fundamentals Preschool-Second Edition* (*CELF-P2*; Wiig, Secord, & Semel, 2006).
- *Communication and Symbolic Behavior Scales* (*CSBS*; Wetherby & Prizant, 1993).
- *Comprehensive Assessment of Spoken Language* (*CASL*; Carrow-Woolfolk, 2008).
- *Early Social Communication Scales* (*ESCS*; Mundy, Delgado, Block, Venezia, Hogan, & Siebert, 2003).
- *Preschool Language Scale-Fifth Edition* (*PLS-5*; Zimmerman et al., 2011).
- *The Rosetti Infant-Toddler Language Scale* (Rosetti, 2005).
- *Test of Pragmatic Language-Second Edition* (*TOPL-2*; Phelps-Terasaki & Phelps-Gunn, 2007).
- *Test of Narrative Language* (*TNL*; Gillam & Pearson, 2004).
- *The SCERTS Assessment Process* found in the *SCERTS Model, Volume I Assessment* (Prizant et al., 2006).

Social Skills

- *Autism Social Skills Profile* (*ASSP*; Bellini, 2006).
- *Pragmatic Language Skills Inventory* (*PLSI*; Gilliam & Miller, 2006).
- *Social Language Development Test-Elementary* (Bowers, Huisingh, LoGiudice, 2008).
- *Social Language Development Test-Adolescent* (Bowers, Huisingh, LoGiudice, 2010).
- *Social Communication Questionnaire* (*SCQ*; Rutter et al., 2003).
- *Social Skill Rating System* (*SSRS*; Gresham & Elliot, 1990).
- *The SCERTS Assessment Process* found in the *SCERTS Model, Volume I Assessment* (Prizant et al., 2006).
- *The Social Responsiveness Scale* (*SRS*; Constantino, 2002).
- *Descriptive Pragmatics Profile* checklist on the *CELF-P2* (Wiig, Secord, & Semel, 2006).
- *Pragmatics Profile* checklist on the *CELF-4* (Semel, Wiig, & Secord, 2003).
- *Pragmatic Protocol* by Prutting and Kirchner (1987).

- The Relationship Development Questionnaire and the Progress Tracking Form from *Relationship Development Intervention with Children, Adolescents and Adults* (*RDI*; Gutstein & Sheely, 2002).

Emergent Literacy

- *Assessment of Literacy and Language* (*ALL*; Lombardino, Lieberman, & Brown, 2005).
- *Emergent Literacy Profile* (*ELP*; Dickinson & Chaney, 1997).
- *Pre-Literacy Rating Scale* on the *CELF-P2* (Wiig, Secord, & Semel, 2006).
- *Preschool Word and Print Awareness* (Justice, Bowles, & Skibbe, 2006).
- *Test of Early Reading Ability-Third Edition* (*TERA-3*; Reid et al., 2001)
- *Test of Preschool Early Literacy* (*TOPEL*; Lonigan, Wagner, & Torgesen, 2007).

Written Language

- *Comprehensive Test of Phonological Processing* (*CTOPP*; Wagner, Torgesen, & Rashotte, 1999).
- *Gray Oral Reading Tests-Fifth Edition* (*GORT-5*; Wiederholt & Bryant, 2012).
- *Process Assessment of the Learner: Diagnostic Assessment for Reading and Writing* (*PAL-II*; Berninger, 2007).
- *Qualitative Reading Inventory-Fifth Edition* (*QRI-5*; Leslie & Caldwell, 2011).
- *Test of Word Reading Efficiency* (*TOWRE*; Torgesen, Wagner, & Rashotte, 1999).
- *Test of Written Spelling-Fourth Edition* (Larsen, Hammill, & Moats, 1999).
- *Woodcock-Johnson Tests of Achievement* (Mather & Woodcock, 2001a).
- *Woodcock-Johnson Tests of Cognitive Abilities* (Mather & Woodcock, 2001b).

Play Skills

- *CSBS* (Wetherby & Prizant, 1993)
- Frameworks and checklists regarding play development found in *Peer Play and the Autism Spectrum: The Art of Guiding Children's Socialization and Imagination* (Wolfberg, 2003), including:
  - Frameworks for Observing Children's Developmental Play Patterns (Table 7–2)
  - Play Questionnaire (pp. 144–147)
  - Profile of Individual Play Development (p. 150)
- Observational assessments and checklists found in *DO-WATCH-LISTEN-SAY* (Quill, 2000), including:
  - *Assessment of Social and Communication Skills for Children with Autism*
  - *Play Interest Survey*
  - *Social Play Task Analysis*

Informational Story

The DVD contains an informational story about what to expect during a communication evaluation. This story in particular was written for a preschool-age child going to receive an evaluation outside of his or her primary natural environment, such as an evaluation conducted in a different therapy room within the child's school or in a therapy center. The reader will also note the story was written for an evaluation that has the caregiver in attendance and participating in the evaluation. Informational stories such as this one can be sent to the child prior to the evaluation as a way to let them know what to expect. This is an excellent tool that frequently prevents problem behavior that might arise because of a child's anxiety about unknown situations. The authors have seen first-hand the difference between children that are informed of what to expect using visual methods versus children who were either not told or the explanation was only given verbally. Children especially appreciate having a picture of the person they will be seeing when they enter the new environment.

Learning Tool

1. How can the SLP be involved with the diagnosis of ASD?

2. Tell how the different types of assessment tools can be beneficial during assessment of children with ASD.

3. Describe the limitations of using standardized assessments with children with ASD.

4. What are some common characteristics of the social communication of children with ASD?

5. How does the development of play relate to language development?

References

American Psychiatric Association. (2000). *Diagnostic and statistical manual of mental disorders* (4th ed., Text rev.). Washington, DC: Author.

American Psychiatric Association. (2013). *Diagnostic and statistical manual of mental disorders* (5th ed.). Washington, DC: Author.

American Speech-Language-Hearing Association. (1993). *Definitions of communication disorders and variations* [Relevant paper]. Retrieved from http://www.asha.org/policy

American Speech-Language-Hearing Association. (2006). *Guidelines for speech-language pathologists in diagnosis, assessment, and treatment of autism spectrum disorders across the life span* [Guidelines]. Retrieved from http://www.asha.org/policy

American Speech-Language-Hearing Association. (2007). *Childhood apraxia of speech* [Position statement]. Retrieved from http://www.asha.org/policy

American Speech-Language-Hearing Association. (2010). *Roles and responsibilities of speech-language pathologists in schools* [Professional issues statement]. Retrieved from http://www.asha.org/policy

Bates, E. (1979). *The emergence of symbols: Cognition and communication in infancy.* New York, NY: Academic Press.

Bates, E., O'Connell, B., & Shore, C. (1987). Language and communication in infancy. In J. Osofsky (Ed.), *Handbook of infant development* (pp. 149–203). New York, NY: John Wiley & Sons.

Bellini, S. (2006). *Building social relationships: A systematic approach to teach social interaction skills to children and adolescents with autism spectrum disorders and other social difficulties.* Shawnee Mission, KS: Autism Asperger Publishing.

Berninger, V. W. (2007). *Process assessment of the learner: Diagnostic assessment for reading and writing II (PAL-II)*. Minneapolis, MN: Pearson.

Beyer, J., & Gammeltoft, L. (1998). *Autism and play.* Philadelphia, PA: Jessica Kingsley.

Bloom, L., & Lahey, M. (1978). *Language development and language disorders.* New York, NY: Wiley.

Bowers, Huisingh, LoGiudice, (2008). *Social Language Development Test-Elementary.* East Moline, IL: LinguiSystems.

Bowers, Huisingh, LoGiudice, (2010). *Social Language Development Test-Adolescent.* East Moline, IL: LinguiSystems.

Bruner, J. (1981). The social context of language acquisition. *Language and Communication, 1,* 155–178.

Carpenter, M., Nagel, K., & Tomasello, M. (1998). Social cognition, joint attention, and communicative competence from 9 to 15 months of age. *Monographs of the Society for Research in Child Development, 63,* 1–143.

Carpenter, M., & Tomasello, M. (2000). Joint attention, cultural learning, and language acquisition: Implications for children with Autism. In A. Wetherby & B. Prizant (Eds.), *Autism spectrum disorders: A transactional developmental perspective* (Vol. 9, pp. 31–54). Baltimore, MD: Paul H. Brookes.

Carrow-Woolfolk, E. (2008). *Comprehensive assessment of spoken language.* Minneapolis, MN: Pearson.

Catts, H. W., Fey, M. E., Zhang, X., & Tomblin, J. B. (1999). Language basis of reading and reading disabilities: Evidence from a longitudinal investigation. *Scientific Studies of Reading, 3,* 331–361.

Catts, H. W., & Kamhi, A. G. (1999). Causes of reading disabilities. In H. W. Catts & A. G. Kamhi (Eds.), *Language and reading disabilities* (pp. 95–127). Boston, MA: Allyn & Bacon.

Centers for Disease Control and Prevention. (2012). http://www.cdc.gov/ncbddd/autism/hcp-recommendations.html

Constantino, J. N. (2002). *The social responsiveness scale.* Los Angeles, CA: Western Psychological Services.

Damico, J., Oller, J., & Tetnowski, J. (1999). Investigating the interobserver reliability of a direct observational language assessment technique. *Advances in Speech-Language Pathology, 1,* 77–94.

Dickinson, D. K., & Chaney, C. (1997). *Emergent literacy profile.* Newton, MA: Education Development Center & Carolyn Chaney.

Ehlers, S., Gillberg, C., & Wing, L. (1999). Autism spectrum screening questionnaire (ASSQ). *Journal of Autism and Developmental Disorders, 29,* 129–141.

Estes, A., Rivera, V., Bryan, M., Cali, P., & Dawson, G. (2011). Discrepancies between academic achievement and intellectual ability in higher-functioning school-aged children with autism spectrum disorder. *Journal of Autism and Developmental Disorders, 41,* 1044–1052.

Filipek, P., Accardo, P., Baranek, G., Cook, E., Dawson, G., Gordon, B., . . . Volkmar, F. R. (1999). The screening and diagnosis of autistic spectrum disorders. *Journal of Autism and Developmental Disorders, 29,* 439–484.

Fox, L., Dunlap, G., & Buschbacher, P. (2000). Understanding and intervening with children's problem behavior: A comprehensive approach. In S. F. Warren & J. Reichle (Series Eds.) and A. M. Wetherby & B. M. Prizant (Vol. Eds.), *Communication and language intervention series: Vol. 9. Autism spectrum disorders: A transactional developmental perspective* (pp. 307–331). Baltimore, MD: Paul H. Brookes.

Garfin, D. G., & Lord, C. (1986). Communication as a social problem in autism. In E. Schoplet & G. B. Mesibov (Eds.), *Social behavior in autism* (pp. 133–152). New York, NY: Plenum Press.

Gilliam, J. E. (2006). *Gilliam Autism Rating Scale, 2nd edition (GARS-2).* Austin, TX: Pro-Ed.

Gilliam, J. E., & Miller, L. (2006). *Pragmatic Language Skills Inventory.* Austin, TX: Pro-Ed.

Gillam, R. B., & Pearson, N. A. (2004). *Test of Narrative Language.* Austin, TX: Pro-Ed.

Gresham, F. M., & Elliot, S. N. (1990). *Social skills rating system manual.* Circle Pines, MN: American Guidance Service.

Grigorenko, E. L., Klin, A., & Volkmar, F. (2003). Annotation: hyperlexia: Disability or superability? *Journal of Child Psychology and Psychiatry, 44,* 1079–1091.

Grossman, R. B., Bemis, R. H., Skwerer, D. P., & Tager-Flusberg, H. (2010). Lexical and affective prosody in children with high-functioning autism. *Journal of Speech Language and Hearing Research, 53,* 778–783.

Gutstein, S. E., & Sheely, R. K. (2002). *Relationship development intervention with young children: Social and emotional development activities for Asperger syndrome, autism, PDD, and NLD.* London, UK: Jessica Kingsley.

Janzen, J. E., & Zenko, C. B. (2012). *Understanding the nature of autism: A guidebook to the autism spectrum disorders* (3rd ed.). San Antonio, TX: Hammill Institute on Disabilities.

Jones, C. R. G., Happe, F., Golden, H., Marsden, A. J. S., Tregay, J., Simonoff, E., . . . Charman, T. Reading and arithmetic in adolescents with autism spectrum disorders: Peaks and dips in attainment. *Neuropsychology, 23,* 718–728.

Justice, L. M., Bowles, R. P., & Skibbe, L. E. (2006). Measuring preschool attainment of print-concept knowledge: A study of typical and at-risk 3- to 5-year-old children using item response theory. *Language, Speech, and Hearing Services in Schools, 37,* 224–235.

Kim, J. A., Szatmari, P., Bryson, S. E., Streiner, D. L., & Wilson, F. J. (2000). The prevalence of anxiety and mood problems among children with autism and Asperger syndrome. *Autism, 4,* 117–132.

Klin, A., Saulnier, C., Tsatsanis, K., & Volkmar, F. (2005). Clinical evaluation in autism spectrum disorders: Psychological assessment within a transdisciplinary framework. In F. Volkmar, R. Paul, A. Klin, & D. Cohen (Eds.), *Handbook of autism and pervasive developmental disorders: Assessment, interventions, and policy* (Vol. 2, pp. 772–798). Hoboken, NJ: Wiley.

Larsen, S. C., Hammill, D. D., & Moats, L. C. (1999). *Test of Written Spelling* (4th ed.). Austin, TX: Pro-Ed.

Leslie, L., & Caldwell, J. S. (2011). *Qualitative Reading Inventory* (5th ed.). Boston, MA: Pearson.

Lombardino, L. J., Lieberman, R. J., & Brown, J. J. C. (2005). *Assessment of Literacy and Language.* San Antonio, TX: PsychCorp.

Lonigan, C. J., Wagner, R. K., & Torgesen, J. K. (2007). *Test of Preschool Early Literacy.* Austin, TX: ProEd.

Lord, C., & Corsello, C. (2005). Diagnostic instruments in autistic spectrum disorders. In F. Volkmar, R. Paul, A. Klin, & D. Cohen (Eds.), *Handbook of autism and pervasive developmental disorders: Assessment, interventions, and policy* (Vol. 2, pp. 730–771). Hoboken, NJ: Wiley.

Lord, C., Rutter, M., DiLavore, P., Risi, S., Gotham, K. R., & Bishop, S. L. (2012). *Autism diagnostic observation schedule* (2nd ed.). Los Angeles, CA: Western Psychological Services.

MacDonald, J. D. (2004). *Communicating partners.* Philadelphia, PA: Jessica Kingsley.

Martin, N. A., & Brownell, R. (2011). *Receptive One-Word Picture Vocabulary Test* (4th ed.). Novato, CA: Academic Therapy.

Mather, N., & Woodcock, R. W. (2001a). *Woodcock-Johnson Tests of Achievement.* Itasca, IL: Riverside.

Mather, N., & Woodcock, R. W. (2001b). *Woodcock-Johnson Tests of Cognitive Abilities.* Itasca, IL: Riverside.

McCune-Nicolich, L., & Carroll, S. (1981). Development of symbolic play: Implications for the language specialist. *Topics in Language Disorders, 2,* 1–15.

McEachin, J. J., Smith, T., & Lovaas, O. I. (1993). Long-term outcome for children with autism who received early intensive behavioral treatment. *American Journal on Mental Retardation, 97,* 359–372.

Ming, X., Brimacombe, M., & Wagner, G. (2007). Prevalence of motor impairment in autism spectrum disorders. *Brain and Development, 29,* 565–570.

Mundy, P., Delgado, C., Block, J., Venezia, M., Hogan, A., & Siebert, J. (2003). *A manual for* the abridged *Early Social Communication Scales (ESCS)*. Coral Gables, FL: University of Miami.

Mundy, P., & Stella, J. (2000). Joint attention, social orienting, and nonverbal communication in Autism. In A. Wetherby & B. Prizant (Eds.), *Autism spectrum disorders: A transactional developmental perspective* (Vol. 9, pp. 55–77). Baltimore, MD: Brookes.

Nation, K., Clarke, P., Wright, B., & Williams, C. (2006). Patterns of reading ability in children with autism spectrum disorder. *Journal of Autism and Developmental Disabilities, 36,* 911–919.

National Research Council. (2001). *Educating children with autism.* Washington, DC: National Academy Press, Committee on Educational Interventions for Children with Autism, Division of Behavioral and Social Sciences and Education.

Norbury, C. & Nation, K. (2011). Understanding variability in reading comprehension in adolescents with autism spectrum disorders: Interactions with language status and decoding skill. *Scientific Studies of Reading, 15*(3), 191–210.

Paul, R. (2005). Assessing communication in autism spectrum disorders. In F. Volkmar, R. Paul, A. Klin, & D. Cohen (Eds.), *Handbook of autism and pervasive developmental disorders: Assessment, interventions, and policy* (Vol. 2, pp. 799–816). Hoboken, NJ: Wiley.

Paul, R. (2007). *Language disorders from infancy through adolescence: Assessment and intervention* (3rd ed.). Mosby Elsevier.

Phelps-Terasaki, D. & Phelps-Gunn, T. (2007). *Test of Pragmatic Language-Second Edition.* Austin, TX: ProEd.

Prizant, B. M., & Rydell, P. J. (1984). Analysis of functions of delayed echolalia in autistic children. *Journal of Speech and Hearing Research, 27,* 183–192.

Prizant, B. M., Wetherby, A. M., Rubin, E., Laurent, A. C., & Rydell, P. J. (2006). *The SCERTS model: A comprehensive educational approach for children with autism spectrum disorders.* Baltimore, MD: Paul Brookes.

Prutting, C. A., & Kirchner, D. M. (1987). A clinical appraisal of the pragmatic aspects of language. *Journal of Speech and Hearing Disorders, 52,* 105–119.

Quill, K. A. (2000). *Do-Watch-Listen-Say.* Baltimore, MD: Paul H. Brookes.

Reid, D. K., Hrasko, W. P., & Hammill, D. D. (2001). *Test of early reading ability* (3rd ed.). Austin, TX: Pro-Ed.

Robbins, D., Fein, D., & Barton, M. (1999). The modified checklist for autism in toddlers (M-CHAT). Retrieved from http://www2.gsu.edu/~psydlr/DianaLRobins/Official_M-CHAT_Website.html

Rosetti, L. (2005). *The Rosetti Infant-Toddler Language Scale.* East Moline, IL: LinguiSystems.

Ruscello, D. M. (2001). *Tests and measurements in speech-language pathology.* Boston, MA: Butterworth-Heinemann.

Rutter, M., Bailey, A., Berument, S. K., Lord, C., & Pickles, A. (2003). *Social communication questionnaire (SCQ).* Los Angeles, CA: Western Psychological Services.

Rutter, M., Le Couteur, A., & Lord, C. (2003). *The Autism Diagnostic Interview–Revised (ADI-R).* Los Angeles, CA: Western Psychological Services.

Schopler, E., Van Bourgondien, M. E., Wellman, G. J., & Love, S. R. (2010). *The childhood autism rating scale* (2nd ed.). Los Angeles, CA: Western Psychological Services.

Semel, E., Wiig, E. H., & Secord, W. A. (2003). *Clinical Evaluation of Language Fundamentals-Fourth Edition.* San Antonio, TX: PsychCorp.

Semel, E., Wiig, E. H., & Secord, W. A. (in press). *Clinical Evaluation of Language Fundamentals-Fifth Edition.* San Antonio, TX: PsychCorp.

Shipley, K. G., & McAfee, J. G. (2004). *Assessment in speech-language pathology.* Clifton Park, NY: Delmar Learning.

Shriberg, L. D., Paul, R., Black, L. M., & Van Santen, J. P. (2011). The hypothesis of apraxia of speech in children with autism spectrum disorder. *Journal of Autism and Developmental Disorders, 41,* 405–426.

Shriberg, L. D., Paul, R., McSweeny, J. L., Klin, A., Cohen, D. J., & Volkmar, F. R. (2001). Speech and prosody characteristics of adolescents and adults with high-functioning autism and Asperger syndrome. *Journal of Speech, Language, and Hearing Research, 44,* 1097–1115.

Shumway, S., & Wetherby, A. M. (2009). Communicative acts of children with autism spectrum disorders in the second year of life. *Journal of Speech, Language, and Hearing Research, 52,* 1139–1156.

Snow, C. E., Burns, M. S., & Griffin, P. (1998). *Preventing reading difficulties in young children.* Washington, DC: National Academy Press.

Stone, W., & Ousley, O. (2004). *Screening tool for autism in two-year olds (STAT).* Nashville, TN: Vanderbilt University.

Tager-Flusberg, H., Paul, R., & Lord, C. (2005). Language and communication in autism. In F. Volkmar, R. Paul, A. Klin, & D. Cohen (Eds.), *Handbook of autism and pervasive developmental disorders* (Vol. 1, pp. 335–364). Hoboken, NJ: Wiley.

Torgesen, J. K., Wagner, R. K., & Rashotte, C. A. (1999). *Test of word reading efficiency.* Austin, TX: Pro-Ed.

Van Steensel, F. J. A., Bögels, S. M., & Perrin, S. (2011). Anxiety disorders in children and adolescents with autistic spectrum disorders: A meta-analysis. *Clinical Child and Family Review, 14,* 302–317.

Wagner, R. K., Torgesen, J. K., & Rashotte, C. A. (1999). *Comprehensive test of phonological processing.* Austin, TX: Pro-Ed.

Westby, C. (2002). Beyond decoding: Critical and dynamic literacy for students with dyslexia, language learning disabilities (LLD), or attention deficit-hyperactivity disorder (ADHD). In K. G. Butler & E. R. Silliman (Eds.), *Speaking, reading and writing in children with language learning disabilities: New paradigms for research and practice* (pp. 73–108). Mahwah, NJ: Erlbaum.

Wetherby, A., & Prizant, B. (1989). The expression of communicative intent: Assessment issues. *Seminars in Speech and Language, 10,* 77–91.

Wetherby, A. M., & Prizant, B. M. (1993). *Communication and symbolic behavior scales.* Chicago, IL: Riverside.

Wetherby, A. M. & Prizant, B. M. (2002). *Communication and Symbolic Behavior Scales Developmental Profile Infant/Toddler Checklist (CSBS-DP).* Baltimore, MD: Paul H Brookes.

Wetherby, A. M., Prizant, B. M., & Schuler, A. L. (2000). Understanding the nature of communication and language impairments. In A. M. Wetherby & B. M. Prizant (Eds.), *Autism spectrum disorders: A transactional developmental perspective* (pp. 109–141). Baltimore, MD: Paul Brookes.

Wiederholt, J. L., & Bryant, B. R. (2012). *Gray oral reading tests* (5th ed.). Austin, TX: Pro-Ed.

Wiig, E. H., Secord, W. A., & Semel, E. (2006). *Clinical Evaluation of Language Fundamentals Preschool-Second Edition.* San Antonio, TX: PsychCorp.

Wolfberg, P. J. (1999). *Play and imagination in children with autism.* New York, NY: Teachers College Press.

Wolfberg, P. J. (2003). *Peer play and the autism spectrum: The art of guiding children's socialization and imagination.* Shawnee Mission, KS: Autism Asperger Publishing.

Wolfberg, P. J. (2009). *Play and imagination in children with autism* (2nd ed.). Columbia, NY: Teachers College Press.

Zimmerman, I. L., Steiner, V. G., & Pond, R. E. (2011). *Preschool language scales* (5th ed.). Bloomington, MN: Pearson.

CHAPTER

4

Intervention Basics

Introduction

This chapter focuses on the topic most SLPs want to know more about: "What do I do in therapy?" Typically, intervention is what SLPs spend the majority of their time doing. As stated in the title of this text, the SLP's goal is to create a balanced intervention and educational plan that will meet the functional needs of the individual child and his or her family. To provide quality intervention, the clinician needs to complete a thorough assessment and then create goals based on the information collected. As mentioned in Chapter 3, assessment can be challenging when working with children on the autism spectrum. Including a variety of assessment types helps provide the necessary pieces to create meaningful treatment and/or educational plans. Quality intervention is based on a solid foundation of understanding what ASD is and how it affects the individual's learning, communication, and behavior. Based on this knowledge and the data collected during assessment about each individual's current levels, strengths, areas of difficulty, and functional needs, the SLP can devise effective intervention strategies to meet the goals set forth on the treatment or educational plan.

The goal of this chapter is to provide information about evidence-based practice for working with the population of children with ASD and their families. Chapter 5 delves further into intervention, specifically with how to provide evidence-based interventions for working with social communication. Chapter 6 then provides more in-depth information about evidence-based practices for working with children to achieve learning and academic outcomes. Finally, Chapter 7 presents real-life cases via case vignettes, video clips, and intervention materials that demonstrate how to apply these concepts into meaningful intervention for children with ASD and their families.

See Chapter 3 for more information on assessment procedures.

According to a publication by the National Research Council (2001), Table 4–1 summarizes what effective interventions for children with autism should follow.

> To order or download the National Research Council (2001) Educating Children with Autism resource, go to: http://www.nap.edu/openbook.php?isbn=0309072697

This chapter uses the recommendations of the National Research Council (2001) as a foundation to describe intervention tools and techniques that work.

Creating Meaningful Goals

The splinter-like developmental profile of most children on the spectrum, along with their unique learning styles, makes standardized assessment and prioritizing treatment goals difficult (Klin, Saulnier, Tsatsanis, & Volkmar, 2005). According to the American Speech-

Table 4–1. Summary of Effective Interventions for Children with Autism

Effective Interventions Should:

- Begin as soon as the individual is suspected of having ASD or related disabilities
- Actively engage the child in learning for a full school day (5 hours), 5 days a week (minimum)
- Be individualized
- Include ongoing assessment of the child's progress
- Teach skills in context (for example, in the places and situations in which they are expected to be used)
- Have a plan for how to teach generalization of skills
- Have a plan for how to teach maintenance of skills
- Include interactions with typically developing children and adults
- Focus on functional, spontaneous communication
- Include social instruction throughout the day
- Focus on play and leisure skills including peers and toys or games
- Include positive approaches to behavior (including functional assessment, functional communication training, and reinforcement of alternative behaviors)

This is a summary of the recommendations the National Research Council (2001, pp. 218–221) endorsed as effective interventions for children with ASD.

Language-Hearing Association (2006a) guidelines, SLPs need to "prioritize learning objectives within natural communication contexts, combining information from a developmental framework, family priorities, functional needs, and learning styles" (5.c.). Using the data gathered during assessment and discussing priorities with the families, individual, and teachers, gives the SLP the information necessary to create functional and meaningful goals that will have the greatest impact on improving the outcomes for children with ASD.

> "Many people ask me, 'What was the big breakthrough that enabled you to lead a successful life?' There was no single break-through. My development was a gradual evolution that had many small but important steps." (p. 1276)
>
> "In my early life, a good education and intervention by age 2½ were crucial." (p. 1285)
>
> —Temple Grandin, a successful adult with ASD, providing a personal perspective of autism (Grandin, 2005)

Knowing what the key goals are for intervention and why they are important is imperative for a clinician to understand, as well as for the individual with whom they are working. Sometimes, therapists forget to discuss targeted goals, rationales, and progress with the most important player in the game, namely, the child. Using a visual support to help explain goals, rationale, and progress helps teach the child how to analyze and monitor their own success. See Figure 4–1 for an example.

Therapy should incorporate meaningful, functional, and motivating activities designed to provide instruction and application practice to the child with ASD. Children with ASD may be motivated by different things than same-age peers, and these motivators may change. Having a solid handle on why you are working on a specific goal allows the clinician to change a specific activity that he or she has planned to target the goal if the current activity is not working. Without a clear understanding of the goal's purpose, it is harder to improvise in the moment to do a different activity targeting the same goal that is more meaningful and motivating to the child.

Having a plan to incorporate each goal in different settings with different communication partners is also vital in an effective intervention plan (National Research Council, 2001; Prizant, Wetherby, Rubin, Laurent, & Rydell, 2006). It is difficult for children with autism to generalize skills, so building in direct time to practice skills outside of the original teaching environment is crucial. An easy way to do this is by involving the parents, caregivers, and/or teachers who interact with the child with autism on a regular basis. This gives the child multiple opportunities to practice any newly acquired skills in different contexts with different people and will increase the likelihood of generalization (Prizant et al., 2006; National Research Council, 2001). Fisher, Frey, and Sax (1999)

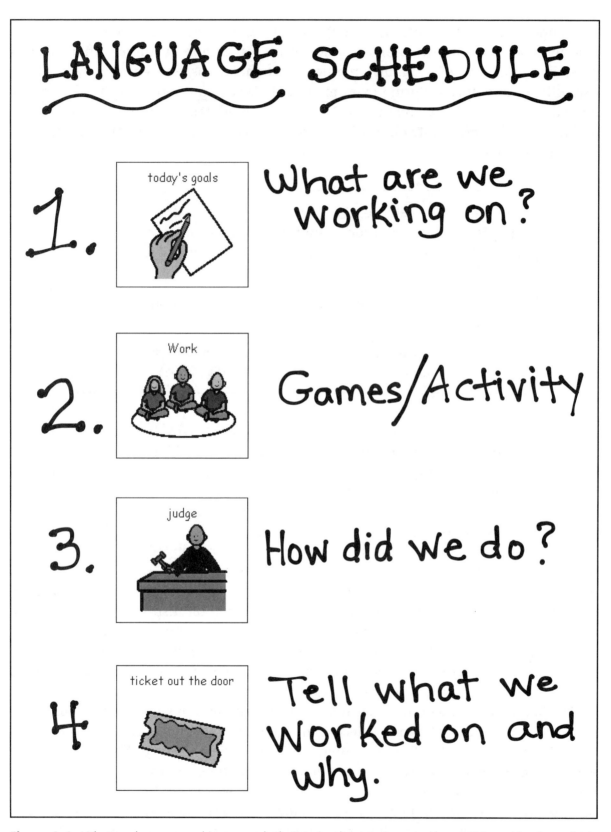

Figure 4–1. What goal are we working on and why? A visual support created by an SLP working in a private practice to promote awareness of therapy goals and self-monitoring of progress. © Brittany Carroll, 2013

created a visual support for the intervention and educational teams to use that helps map out when and where it makes the most sense to target each goal, called an Infused Skills Grid. This easy-to-use grid helps the adults think and plan what goals can and should be targeted during different times and in different settings (See Figure 4–2 for a sample Infused Skills Grid).

As with any intervention, developing a reliable way to track progress is important but often challenging when working with kids on the autism spectrum. Build in a user-friendly way to collect meaningful data, so all parties who are working on the goal can report progress.

IEP and Treatment Plan Goals

IEP stands for Individualized Education Program and is a document created for students who are eligible for special education services in the public school system. IEPs are derived from the Individuals with Disabilities Education Act (IDEA) revised in 2004. An SLP working in the school system will be a part of the IEP team and be required to develop goals for communication and participate in IEP meetings. The meetings are set up for the entire educational team (teachers, therapists, administrators, families) to gather and discuss each student's current educational support needs and develop a plan that outlines goals and supports that target the student's needs. The IEP team must meet at least once a year to update goals and current levels of performance and discuss any changes that need to be made. The IEP team can meet as often as the team deems necessary, but they have to meet at least once per year.

There are critical components to include when writing goals for an IEP. All goals need to include present level of performance followed by what the goal will target and what parameter defines mastery of each goal. An IEP must include a broad annual goal followed by more specific benchmarks or objectives that will target the skill(s) identified in the annual goal. For each objective, the SLP needs to identify how he or she will measure progress so data can be collected regularly and reported once every nine weeks. Additionally, SLPs in 45 states are now being called on to integrate the Common Core State Standards within their interventions and ensure that children with disabilities are provided opportunities to be exposed to the same standard of education as typically developing children (Common Core State Standards Initiative, 2012). The American Speech-Language Hearing Association provides an overview to assist SLPs with incorporating these standards into educational plans.

See the following link for an overview of the Common Core State Standards for the SLP:
http://www.asha.org/SLP/schools/Common-Core-State-Standards.htm

Filled out by: Heather Caseres and Desiree Williams –IEP Planning Goals

Infused Skills

1. Acknowledge interaction by classmate verbally
2. Work with peers in small group without stereotypic behavior
3. Follow instructions from classmates
4. Verbally express choice
5. Express need for wait time
6. Verbally initiate communication with questions

Infused Skills Grid

Student Name: M	General Teacher: __
Age: 13 Grade: 7th	Special Ed. Teacher: _____

Date: _____ October 15, 2012 _____   **IEP Goals / Infused Skills**

Activities / Subjects	1	2	3	4	5	6			
Arrival	X				X				
English	X	X	X	X	X	X			
Math	X		X	X	X	X			
Lunch	X		X	X	X	X			
Social Studies/History	X	X	X	X	X	X			
Science	X	X	X	X	X	X			
Specials: Art/PE/Music	X	X	X	X	X	X			
ESE Class	X	X	X	X	X	X			
Dismissal	X			X	X				
Check here if the infused skill has been identified by: — Family	X	X			X	X			
Student		X	X	X	X	X			
Peers	X	X	X	X	X	X			
School	X	X	X	X	X				

From: Fisher, D., Frey, N., and Sax, C. (1999). *Inclusive elementary schools: Recipes for success*. Colorado Springs, CO: PEAK Parent Center, Inc.

Figure 4–2. Infused Skills Grid (Fisher et al., 1999). Here is an example of a completed Infused Skills Grid for a seventh-grade student with autism.

Here is one example of a goal with benchmarks (National Association of Special Education Teachers, 2012):

Annual Goal: _____ will demonstrate social communication skills as measured by the benchmarks listed below.

   a. _____ will initiate communicative interactions with others 4 out of 5 opportunities to do so.

   b. _____ will initiate communicative interactions with others by asking questions 4 out of 5 opportunities to do so.

   c. _____ will engage in conversational turn-taking with others across 3 to 4 conversational turns, 4 out of 5 opportunities to do so (topics initiated by self or others).

The National Research Council (2001) summarized what educational goals should target. These recommendations can easily be used in a clinical setting, as well as to help prioritize effective treatment goals. As you can see from Table 4–2, most of the items listed could fall under the scope of practice of the SLP (with a few exceptions). Use the list in Table 4–2 and the data you gather from each student's assessment to guide your goal-writing efforts.

> For more information on IDEA, IEPs, and goal writing and data tracking, see:
>
> http://idea.ed.gov/explore/home
>
> http://www.wrightslaw.com/info/iep.index.htm
>
> http://www.speakingofspeech.com/IEP_Goal_Bank.html
>
> http://specialed.about.com/od/iep/a/iepGoalWriting.htm
>
> http://www.asha.org/uploadedFiles/Writing-Measurable-Goals-and-Objectives.pdf#search=%22writing%22

Writing goals for a clinical treatment plan will vary depending on the requirements of each setting, including those of third-party payers. However, the basic concept of writing treatment goals remains. Each goal needs to identify: (1) what skills will be targeted, (2) in what context the skill will be observed, (3) what supports will be used, (4) what criteria will be used to measure the progress, and (5) a description of the functional rationale. Depending on the setting, the data collection and reporting time frame and format may vary. Different insurance companies, clinics, or federal programs (e.g., Medicaid) have specific requirements regarding how data is recorded and reported and how often. It is the clinician's responsibility to find out the expectations and procedures each setting requires for monitoring treatment goals and data reporting.

Table 4–2. Appropriate Educational Goals

Goals Should Help Develop:

- Functional, spontaneous communication using verbal language or alternative modes of communication (a way for the individual to tell others what he wants, thinks, sees, feels, etc.)

- Receptive language (a way for the person to understand us)

- Increased engagement with other people

- Social skills

- Flexibility

- Motor skills used for age-appropriate, functional activities

- Cognitive skills and academic skills

- Replacement of problem behaviors with more appropriate behaviors

- Independent organizational skills and other behaviors needed for success in regular education classrooms

This is a summary of the priority education goals the National Research Council (2001, pp. 218–221) recommended for students with ASD.

Regardless of the setting, creating meaningful and functional therapy goals is an important step down the path to quality intervention. Using data from various types of assessment and input from the family, individuals, and other providers is the best way to create an effective therapy plan. Each goal should target skills that will have the most impact on positive outcomes for the individuals with autism at home, in the community, and in learning environments. Focusing therapy goals on a variety of areas affected by ASD will help create a balanced intervention approach. Working on one specific area of language at a time can make generalization even slower. Try to incorporate various goals into each session so the children with ASD can start to see and experience how socialization and communication are intricately woven together and allow them more opportunities to practice a variety of skills. Remember to include the families, educators, and other professionals in your therapy plan so that the child with autism has multiple partners and settings to practice their new skills (National Research Council, 2001; Prizant et al., 2006).

Effective Intervention: Key Concepts

According to Table 4–1, the National Research Council (2001) summarized the basic aspects of effective interventions for children with autism. Using their findings, the rest of this chapter outlines basic intervention techniques that follow *best practice* guidelines for children on the autism spectrum.

Early Intervention

The first point says to begin intervention as soon as a child is suspected of having ASD or other disabilities. Ideally, this is done through early intervention when the child is between the ages of zero to three years old. Research shows that early intervention improves outcomes for children with ASD (Mundy & Burnette, 2005; Mundy & Neal, 2001). The entire premise of early intervention is based on the concept of neural plasticity and brain development (Dawson & Zanolli, 2003). When children are young (zero to three years), their brain cells are still developing and are extremely plastic, meaning easily changed. Therefore, the earlier children who are showing signs of autism are identified, the faster they can be placed in intensive, early intervention that will target the areas of development that are delayed (Dawson & Zanolli, 2003; Mundy & Burnette, 2005). However, this does not mean that if a child does not get early intervention that they will not be able to make progress. Early intervention is ideal because of the developing and plastic nature of the brain, but neural plasticity exists in brains young and old (Stiles, 2000). Parents often feel guilty or a sense of doom if their child did not receive early intervention services, but intervention at any age is better than no intervention at all (Stiles, 2000).

Teach Skills in Context

The concepts involved in early intervention are applicable to children on the autism spectrum throughout the lifespan, namely, remain child-focused, family-centered, and strive for meaningful outcomes. These concepts fall in line with the recommendations set forth by the National Research Council (2001) and the American Speech-Language-Hearing Association (2006a, 2008). According to American Speech-Language-Hearing Association policy (2008), the role of the SLP working in early intervention is based on the following guiding principles:

- Services are family-centered and culturally and linguistically responsive.
- Services are developmentally supportive and promote children's participation in their natural environments.
- Services are comprehensive, coordinated, and team-based.
- Services are based on the highest quality evidence that is available.

> See Case Study A discussed in Chapter 7. The materials on the accompanying DVD demonstrate the child's parent describing her primary concerns (A–1) and the ways that the parent's concerns were targeted (A–2 through A–8).

The experts agree that utilizing a naturalistic, child-directed, and family-centered intervention technique is the most effective form of intervention for young children with

ASD (National Research Council, 2001). Some specific examples of child-directed strategies include:

- Follow the child's lead. Incorporate what they are already doing into your therapy session. You are more likely to gain and maintain their attention if you join in on what they are already focused (Sussman, 1999).

- Create an environment that is filled with natural reasons to communicate, or communicative temptations (Wetherby & Prizant, 1989). Incidental teaching is an approach often used to create natural learning opportunities (McGee, Morrier, & Daly, 1999).

- Imitate what the child does. Joining in with what they are doing by mimicking them often gets their attention and provides an opening into their world (Sussman, 1999).

- Interpret what the child says or is trying to say. We often tell parents to "narrate" their child's world to provide verbal models and language content to associate with different experiences (Sussman, 1999). Carpenter and Tomasello (2000) reviewed research findings indicating a correlation between caregivers' modeling of language that follows the child's attentional focus and related increases in these children's language comprehension and expression during early language development. Children with ASD have particular difficulty shifting attention (Akshoomoff, 2000) and establishing joint attention (Carpenter & Tomasello, 2000). Therefore, children with ASD need language modeling that follows their lead to maximize potential opportunities for shared reference. Build on what they are already focused on, so that the child does not have to shift their attention toward your preferred target (Landry & Bryson, 2004).

- Prompt when necessary. If the child is not able to complete the task independently, using a least-to-most prompting hierarchy, simultaneous prompting and graduated guidance have all been proven effective for children on the spectrum (Neitzel & Wolery, 2009). A prompt by definition is any assistance given to the learner to help them complete any given task. The least-to-most prompts, often called the system of least prompts, utilizes at least three levels of prompts, starting with zero assistance then gradually adding support (Neitzel & Wolery, 2009). Prompts are added in the system of least prompts in the following order: gestural, verbal, visual, model, and physical (Neitzel & Wolery, 2009). Simultaneous prompting is when you present the task and give a prompt immediately to ensure success, to essentially act as a model to show how to complete the given task successfully. The next time the task is presented, the prompt is not given immediately to see if the child can do it independently (Neitzel & Wolery, 2009). Graduated guidance is similar in that when the task is first presented, a prompt is automatically given. As the child starts to show proficiency, the clinician must use clinical judgment to decide when to remove the prompt (Neitzel & Wolery, 2009).

Intensity of Intervention

The National Research Council (2001) report states that children with autism should be actively engaged (e.g., learning) for at least 25 hours per week. This can be during school, therapy sessions, at home or in the community working with caregivers. The only way to ensure 25 quality, actively engaged hours of instruction is to enlist the help of all parties: therapists, teachers, parents, caregivers, peers, and so forth. Communicating with all providers and team members regarding the goals and strategies the child is working on is key to making the most of the 25 hours. Each child with autism is unique; therefore, make sure goals and therapy plans are tailored to the individual needs of the child.

The SCERTS model utilizes a framework for intervention focusing on *S*ocial *C*ommunication (SC), *E*motional *R*egulation (ER), and *T*ransactional *S*upports (TS; Prizant et al., 2006). Within the assessment phase of the SCERTS model, an Activity Planning Form is used to guide the team to look at all of the goals within the three main categories (SC, ER, TS) and map out how each goal or objective can be woven into the child's daily activities. This method of actively planning how to infuse goals throughout various times, environments, and activities is one example of how a team can ensure that their intervention plan follows the above recommendation of creating 25 quality hours of intervention in multiple contexts.

Plan for Generalization and Maintenance

A common theme repeated throughout this chapter is to plan for generalization and practice skills in multiple environments with different people. This goes back to the bottom layer of the balanced intervention pyramid, understanding the underlying aspects of ASD. One of the features of ASD is that children often learn new things in a routine and remember it exactly the way it was taught the first time. Being able to apply the new skill in a novel setting is not automatic for children with autism, hence the need to build in a plan for generalization (Janzen & Zenko, 2012). It can be difficult to create different contexts or environments to practice generalization in a clinical or school setting. Introducing new people as interaction partners can provide different practice contexts.

Recruiting other people to carry out generalizations should start with the family. Educate the caregivers on the concepts you are trying to teach and model ways for them to practice at home or in the community. Research has demonstrated that educating caregivers results in gains for the child with ASD (National Research Council, 2001; Vismara, Colombi, & Rogers, 2009). Caregivers are with their children longer than any therapist, so it is imperative to see the caregivers as an extension of your therapeutic arms. This also fulfills the recommendation of family-centered intervention. The American Speech-Language-Hearing Association practice policy documents support this, noting that the role of the SLP involves not only providing direct service, but also working and collaborating with families and other professionals working with children with ASD (American Speech-Language-Hearing Association, 2006a).

Depending on the dynamics between the caregivers, therapist, and child, some clinicians have specified times at the beginning or end of therapy that is dedicated to incorporating caregivers in the session. Give the caregivers one task to work on each week so they are not overwhelmed with the additional task to their already hectic lives. Provide home practice activities that are infused into activities that already occur. These activities can be written down in a "home practice sheet" that explains and summarizes to caregivers what they are supposed to work on and key strategies to try. It may be helpful to the family to have a place to keep track of what happened when they practiced at home, including any questions they might have.

Teaching parents and caregivers may seem like a daunting task, but it is worth the effort (Mahoney & Wiggers, 2007). Utilize resources that are available and written just for parents. One resource, *More Than Words: A Guide to Helping Parents Promote Communication and Social Skills in Children with Autism Spectrum Disorder* (Sussman, 1999), was written for parents and uses easy to understand language and illustrations. The *More Than Words* book or program uses fun acronyms and other mnemonics to help parents remember key techniques to use when communicating with their children on the autism spectrum. For example, the first lesson teaches parents to "OWL: Observe, Wait and Listen." This concept may seem rudimentary to the SLP, but parents often do not realize how important it is to *observe* from the child's level (get down on the floor) and wait for them to process your request (Sussman, 1999).

> For more information on all the programs and products from the Hanen Centre go to their website: http://www.hanen.org

Focus on Functional, Spontaneous Communication

Functional and spontaneous are two imperative concepts when it comes to communication intervention for children on the autism spectrum. The translation of the word functional in speech-language terminology often means the SLP needs to look over the information collected during assessment, so he or she can see what functions of language the child uses and what functions are missing. Based on this information, the SLP has specific language functions to target during therapy.

The intended meaning of the word functional in the National Research Council (2001) publication refers to the more universal definition of the word functional, meaning useful. Individuals with ASD need to have a way to communicate their basic wants, needs, ideas, and desires in a way that others understand. If an individual does not have a way to effectively communicate, they are more prone to use their behavior, often considered *inappropriate,* to express what they are trying to say.

It is up to the SLP to lead the charge to find an effective mode of communication for the individual with ASD. As previously discussed, the autism spectrum is broad and individuals' communication abilities vary greatly. Some children with autism do not use words or speech to communicate. Therefore, an augmentative or alternative communication (AAC) system needs to be developed to meet the individual's communication needs. The AAC method can range from using objects, pictures, sign language, or voice-output devices, depending on what the team decides is the best route for each child.

> See Chapters 5 and 6 for more information about AAC.

Children with ASD who can and do speak may need AAC supports as well. Just because a child speaks, does not mean they always understand everything they hear. When children with ASD are under stress or in unfamiliar situations, their ability to use their words is often compromised (Hodgden, 1996, 1999). Be cognizant of potential expressive and receptive language difficulties even in the children with ASD who talk.

The reference to spontaneous language goes hand-in-hand with functionality. Children with ASD often are *responders*; meaning, they can answer questions or respond when asked but are not always good at initiating interactions. Responding is easier than initiating, and children on the spectrum often fall victim to a hoard of *quizzing* adults (Sussman, 1999). Therefore, they do not always get ample opportunities to practice initiating before an adult or peer starts an interaction. It is imperative to ensure that intervention focuses on initiation of communication as well as responding.

Target Social Instruction with Peers

Social understanding is one of the hallmark areas of difficulty for individuals on the autism spectrum and has a profound impact on several facets of their day-to-day success (Arick, Krug, Fullerton, Loos, & Falco, 2005; Rao, Beidel, & Murray, 2008; Winner & Crooke, 2011). Knowing how to play and get along with others are skills children learn at a young age. Through their natural social experiences, typically developing children's play skills, social interaction, and communication skills evolve without the need for direct instruction. In contrast, children on the autism spectrum need direct instruction on the basic social interaction skills that come naturally to most children, so they can learn to play and socialize successfully.

Teaching children with autism the social nuances required to play, converse, and maintain relationships is an ongoing process. Knowing where to begin is often the biggest hurdle. Therefore, the only way to know where to begin is to assess the child's current social profile that includes his or her strengths, weaknesses, and any gaps in *typical* social development. Bellini (2006, pp. 68–71) lists several social assessments available to help the clinician gauge where to start with social instruction.

Social interaction is not a discrete skill, so transferring any of the ideas taught in a direct fashion requires practice in a multitude of environments with a variety of partners.

It is important to understand the difference between declarative knowledge and procedural knowledge, especially when you are working with a child or adolescent with ASD. According to the description of ASD and the learning strengths and weaknesses in Chapter 2 (Table 2–1), children with autism are usually good at taking in large chunks of information and remembering them for a long time. If the child with autism can repeat the social skill or rule you are working on, that only demonstrates they have acquired the declarative knowledge of the skill. This does not mean they understand the procedural knowledge or how to actually use, execute, or apply the skill in a meaningful setting (Bellini, 2006). To alter the cliché, practice makes perfect; when teaching social skills to children with autism, practice is the only way to make the skills meaningful and acquire the necessary procedural knowledge. Therefore, the recommendations to "include social instruction throughout the day, include interaction with typically developing peers and to teach (directly) play and leisure skills" make sense (National Research Council, 2001).

The Importance of Play

Understanding the significance and connection between the development of play skills and communication and how it affects children on the autism spectrum is paramount. As discussed in Chapters 1 and 3, play skills can be viewed from two developmental continuums: both in the level of symbolism demonstrated and how the play involves others socially (Quill, 2000; Wolfberg, 2009). We know from the DSM-IV-TR that children with ASD may express "lack of varied, spontaneous make-believe play or social imitative play appropriate to developmental level" (American Psychiatric Association, 2000, p. 75). Therefore, assessing play skills on both continuums and incorporating intervention goals that target any gaps in play development is necessary.

For intervention, an SLP needs to directly teach appropriate play skills by creating an engaging environment with a variety of toys that progressively span the symbolic continuum. Children with ASD often play with toys in unconventional ways. For example, a child with ASD may take a toy truck and flip it over to spin the wheels instead of driving it around the rug like his or her peers. The SLP needs to model how to play with a truck by rolling it on the ground and commenting on what he or she is doing. As play skills move away from constructive play and toward symbolic play, children with ASD need to be taught how to *pretend* by modeling and role playing (Wolfberg, 2009).

Although play remains an area of difficulty for children with ASD, it is a misconception that children with ASD do not seek social interaction or will not develop play skills. Children with ASD often need explicit instruction in the area of imaginative play and in developing play skills that allow for creativity and flexibility (Quill, 2000). The social evolution of play starts with solitary play, moves to parallel play, and ends with cooperative play (Wolfberg, 2009). It is important to assess and observe where the child's current level of social play is before creating intervention goals to target growth. The SLP will assist with creating situations for the child to learn the next step through graduated play guidance (Wolfberg, 2009) that provides experiences designed for the child's zone of proximal development (ZPD; Vygotsky, 1978). For instance, if a child with ASD is only interested in solitary play and is not showing signs of noticing others around him or her, the next progression is to guide the child to orient to peers by giving the interesting toys to nearby peers and then the clinician talks aloud about what the children are doing (*orienting* play guidance strategy noted in Wolfberg, 2009). The SLP helps the child gradually develop skills leading toward cooperative, pretend play (Quill, 2000; Wolfberg, 2009). Additional strategies recommended for play intervention by Wolfberg (2009) include: supporting the child's play initiations, scaffolding the child's play level with graduated cues according to the child's performance, and providing support to the social communication that occurs with peers in the context of play (e.g., help the child initiate play with peers, respond to peers, join in ongoing exchanges, etc.). Overall, understanding both dimensions of play development and how they relate to later social communication success is key to developing meaningful intervention plans in order to structure therapy in the child's ZPD.

Include Positive Approaches to Behavior

It is important for the clinician to utilize positive behavior support techniques (discussed in detail in Chapter 2). Many therapists have expressed their number one concern about working with children with ASD is that problem behaviors interfere with achieving intervention outcomes. Susan Stokes (2001) provides a metaphor of an iceberg for understanding behavior in autism. The *challenging behaviors* that are visible are referred to as the "tip of the iceberg" behaviors. In order to understand why the behavior is occurring, you have to look under the surface to see all of the factors that may be contributing to the visible behavior (Figure 4–3).

The iceberg analogy is another way of illustrating the concept of the balanced intervention pyramid (Figure 4–4). They both are built around the premise that in order to understand why a person with autism is behaving a certain way, you have to start by reflecting on what ASD is and how it affects each individual. The sensory processing differences in individuals with autism are one of the first areas to consider when *challenging* behaviors occur.

We know from Chapters 1 and 2 that children with autism often process sensory information differently. Understanding their sensory profiles is vital to the success of any intervention program because the clinician can try to prevent challenging behaviors that might occur due to sensory differences. Knowing how each child reacts when he or she experiences various sensory stimuli is an important part of any clinicians' ongoing assessment. Certain senses can be hypersensitive, meaning it does not take much input for it to register or hyposensitive, where it takes an intense amount of input for the child to even register the stimuli (Ayers, 1979). Among clinicians, you often hear the term *sensory-seekers* versus *sensory-avoiders* (Ayers, 1979; Kranowitz, 2005). If a child is a *sensory-seeker*, it means that they are hyposensitive and are seeking more input for it to make sense to their brain. On the contrary, when children are described as *sensory-avoiders,* that particular sense or input channel is hypersensitive and needs very minimal input to register and often feel overwhelmed (Ayers, 1979; Kranowitz, 2005).

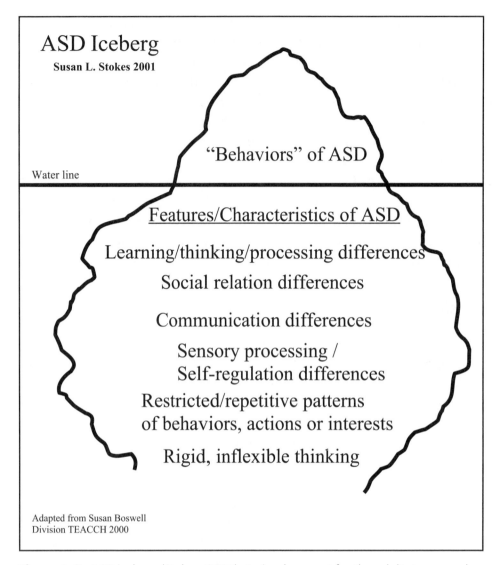

Figure 4–3. ASD iceberg (Stokes, 2001). A visual support for the adults to remember all of the aspects of ASD that lie underneath the iceberg that could be contributing to the behaviors seen on the surface.

A child can present with a mixed sensory profile, meaning be both hypo- and hypersensitive to different sensory input. For example, a child who covers his or her ears or has to wear headphones to keep the auditory information around him or her from hurting is hypersensitive to auditory input, or is a *sensory-avoider* when it comes to auditory stimuli. That same child may also seek hugs, like to wear compression clothing or sit in beanbags, illustrating he or she is hyposensitive to touch and seeks out more input.

As stated in Chapter 2, all individuals have a range of their *optimal level of stress* that keeps them alert enough to pay attention and take in new information, but not too stressed to comprehend (Klinger & Dawson, 1992). Unfortunately, individuals with autism tend to have a narrower window of optimal stress levels for learning (Klinger & Dawson, 1992). The SCERTS model refers to this narrow window as an "optimal arousal level" or when individuals are "available to learn" (Prizant et al., 2006). The Alert Program

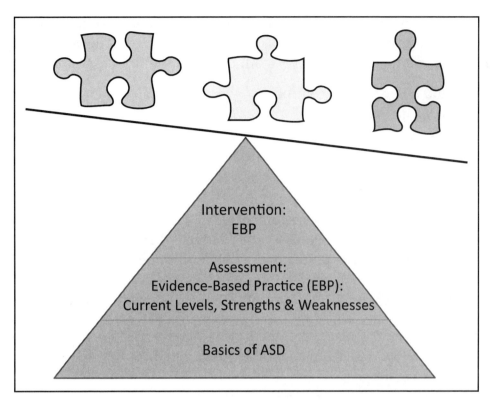

Figure 4–4. Balanced instruction pyramid.

(Williams & Shellenberger, 1996) makes this abstract concept of *optimal arousal* into a child-friendly metaphor of keeping their engine (their brain and body/arousal levels) in the just right speed. Despite the differing terminology, both programs emphasize the fact that no new learning can take place until the child is just right, available to learn, or at their optimal arousal levels.

See http://alertprogram.com and http://scerts.com for more information.

Therefore, clinicians need to read the child's signals of distress or boredom and provide strategies or environmental modifications to help bring the child back to a state where they can take in information. The SCERTS model states very clearly to address the child's emotional regulation (ER) state and goals *first* so that the child is available to learn *before* targeting any other communication, academic, or social goals in order to achieve success. This follows the research that states that the human body is not capable of learning and retaining new skills if it is outside the optimal stress level window required for learning (Klinger & Dawson, 1992).

The ultimate goal for any child on the autism spectrum is to be able to recognize their arousal level and be able to adjust their own *engine speed* so he or she can remain in control. This abstract concept is difficult for children on the autism spectrum and often needs to be directly taught. Buron and Curtis (2012) developed a resource called *The Incred-*

ible 5-Point Scale that uses a numbered scale from 1 to 5 to help concretely and visually depict different levels of stress, frustration, anxiety, and so forth. The original format uses the following descriptors for Levels 1 to 5, but can be customized to fit each child:

5 = This could make me lose control.

4 = This can really upset me.

3 = This can make me nervous.

2 = This sometimes bothers me.

1 = This never bothers me.

This visual scale that incorporates numbers to represent different levels of self-control, utilizes the visual learning strength associated with children on the spectrum, and helps identify what situations create dysregulation while outlining strategies at each level to help return to equilibrium. For more information and ideas on how to use *The Incredible 5-Point Scale* (Buron & Curtis, 2012), go to http://www.5pointscale.com.

> See Case Study C–7 on the DVD for an example of a personalized 5-point scale.

Visually depicted information, especially new concepts, are easier for most individuals with ASD to comprehend (Hodgden, 1996, 1999; Janzen & Zenko, 2012). Presenting information in both an auditory and visual format increases the likelihood of understanding and decreases stress. The research has shown that using visual schedules can teach children with autism to independently transition from one activity to the next, reduce challenging behaviors, and decrease dependence on verbal prompting (National Autism Center, 2009).

> See Case Study A–4 through A–6 on the DVD for examples of how visual supports make transitions easier.

One first-hand account of how important visuals are to individuals with autism is in Temple Grandin's book, *Thinking in Pictures: My Life with Autism* (2006). The first chapter starts out with this quote:

> I think in pictures. Words are like a second language to me. I translate both spoken and written words into full-color movies, complete with sound, which run like a VCR tape in my head. When somebody speaks to me, his words are instantly translated into pictures. (p. 3)

While teaching a parent-training series that emphasized the importance of utilizing visual supports to help children learn and communicate, one author coined a phrase after saying it over and over again. "Cathy's rule" states, "If you say it, show it." These six words helped parents remember and alter their own communication interactions to include some form of visual cue.

Models of Intervention

The above recommendations describe *what* intervention should target. The next question that needs to be answered is *how* to execute the interventions. According to the American Speech-Language-Hearing Association (2006a), there are three basic models of service-delivery for SLPs: pull-out, push-in, or classroom/community-based intervention and consultation. The pull-out model involves removing the child from their current environment and working on goals in a separate location, usually the SLP's therapy room or classroom. When SLPs push-in to deliver services, they bring their materials and work on the communication goals in the child's classroom or other environment outside the therapy room. If you are a clinic-based SLP, the push-in model is more difficult because of logistics, but not impossible. However, providing consultation, the last type of service-delivery model, is not only possible, but also imperative regardless of your location. The consultation model does not involve working directly with the child; instead it entails working with all the professionals who are responsible for the child's intervention and education. Consultation allows the SLP to coordinate with the child's teachers, caregivers, and other providers. This collaboration between SLP and other members of the intervention team provides the opportunity to share goals and techniques that each party is working on, so that carryover and generalization in all environments are more likely (American Speech-Language-Hearing Association, 2006a, 2006b; Diehl, 2003).

A one-on-one or small group setting is recommended when providing direct instruction of new skills (National Autism Center, 2009; National Research Council, 2001). In order to ensure generalization and maintenance of any newly taught skills, the clinician must take the child with ASD into the contexts where the skills will be used and provide coaching and modeling as the child tries to apply the new skills (push-in or classroom/community-based model; Cirrin & Penner, 1995). Finally, to maintain the skill over time, the SLP needs to inform, educate, and enlist the other members of the intervention team, who are with the child all the time, to help facilitate the mastery of each skill (National Autism Center, 2009; National Research Council, 2001). Therefore, using all models of service-delivery are necessary for a successful intervention plan that adheres to evidence-based practices (American Speech-Language-Hearing Association, 2006a, 2006b; Cirrin & Penner, 1995; Diehl, 2003; Ehren, 2002; National Autism Center, 2009; National Research Council, 2001).

How to Select the Best Evidence-Based Practice Approach

There are several intervention strategies to choose from, and it is important to know the evidence regarding efficacy for each approach. The National Standards Report (National Autism Center, 2009) reviewed the level of scientific evidence behind several common educational and behavioral approaches commonly used to treat individuals with autism. The report determined if the treatment effects were: (a) beneficial, (b) ineffective, (c) adverse, or (d) unknown (National Autism Center, 2009, p. 24). Based on the level, amount, and quality of the research findings, the National Autism Center report assigns each intervention or treatment a label of: (a) established, (b) emerging, (c) unestablished, or (d) ineffective/harmful (National Autism Center, 2009, p. 32).

> To read the entire National Standards Report, go to: http://www
> .nationalautismcenter.org/pdf/NAC%20Standards%20Report.pdf

It's often difficult to collect reliable data on different intervention techniques based on the abstract concepts targeted. Always check to see if the approach is considered an established evidence-based practice (EBP). If the approach is new or does not have a significant evidence base, you need to use your best clinical judgment before using and ask yourself:

Does this intervention target the core deficits of ASD?

Does it have a clear way to assess the child's current levels, strengths, and weaknesses?

Does the approach make broad claims without sufficient evidence?

Does the intervention make sense and target areas the child needs to improve?

Recognizing that the efficacy data is lacking in the area of autism treatments, the National Standard Report (National Autism Center, 2009, pp. 77–78) provides four domains to consider when determining whether or not to use a specific intervention technique.

1. Research Findings: What does the research say about the approach?
2. Professional Judgment: Based on your clinical experience and data, is the approach proving effective?
3. Values and Preferences: Does the approach satisfy the goals and ideals of the parents, the provider (you), and the individual on the autism spectrum?
4. Capacity: Do you have proper training in the approach or is it available? Do you have adequate resources to carry out the approach? Is there a way to clearly track the fidelity of the approach?

As long as you follow the above guidelines, implementing an intervention approach that does not have extensive efficacy data is within the guidelines of best practices. However, keeping your own data is even more critical when utilizing *unproven* approaches. The goal of all intervention is to provide positive outcomes without harming the individual or their family. Proceed with caution when the empirical evidence is lacking and form solid clinical decisions based on data you collect.

Summary: Ten Basic Intervention Tips to Remember

Based on the evidence collected by the National Research Council (2001), this chapter outlined several basic intervention recommendations for children on the autism spectrum. The following is a list of the top ten intervention tips to remember.

1. Always go back and review what ASD is and how it affects learning and behavior. Remember that each child with ASD is unique. Establish how ASD affects each individual and customize your intervention plan accordingly.

2. Always start by assessing the child's *E*motion *R*egulation (**ER** from SCERTS model) state. If the child is not well regulated, implement strategies to help bring them back to just right (Alert Program) speed before trying to teach any new information.

3. Always ask yourself, "What goal are we working on and why?," so you always have a clear understanding of the desired outcome. This will allow you to improvise and change activities quickly while targeting the same goal.

4. Remember to follow the child's lead. Get down on their level and observe, wait, and listen (OWL; Sussman, 1999). Being face-to-face improves your chances of catching and maintaining their attention.

5. Incorporate their interest areas into your therapy plan. Use these interests to your advantage. Children with ASD are more likely to engage and pay attention if you are using their favorite things.

6. Listen to what the child with autism is trying to say or what their behavior is trying to say, and adapt accordingly. Remember that behavior is communication, and it is an outward expression of an inward state. Take data to figure out why the behavior is happening and come up with equally effective, more acceptable replacement behaviors.

7. Generalization is difficult for children on the autism spectrum. Be sure to plan for opportunities to practice any new skills in a variety of environments with a variety of people.

8. Be sure each child with ASD has a functional way to communicate his or her wants, needs, and ideas. If children do not have a way to communicate effectively, they will probably exhibit challenging behaviors. Remember to use visual supports to improve both expressive and receptive language by following Cathy's rule, "If you say it, show it."

9. Always take data to support and monitor each intervention goal. This is the only way to know if an intervention is working.

10. Take time to develop a strong team relationship. Collaboration with all individuals who support a child with ASD is the key to success.

Learning Tool

1. Name five effective interventions outlined by the National Research Council (2001).

2. What should always be included in any treatment goal?

3. Why is teaching skills in context important to children with ASD?

References

Akshoomoff, N. (2000). Neurological underpinnings of autism. In A. Wetherby & B. Prizant (Eds.), *Autism spectrum disorders: A transactional developmental perspective* (Vol. 9, pp. 167–190). Baltimore, MD: Paul H. Brookes.

American Psychiatric Association. (2000). *Diagnostic and statistical manual of mental disorders* (4th ed., Text rev.). Washington, DC: Author.

American Speech-Language-Hearing Association. (2006a). *Guidelines for speech-language pathologists in diagnosis, assessment, and treatment of autism spectrum disorders across the life span* [Guidelines]. Retrieved from http://www.asha.org/policy

American Speech-Language-Hearing Association. (2006b). *Knowledge and skills needed by speech-language pathologists for diagnosis, assessment, and treatment of autism spectrum disorders across the life span* [Knowledge and skills]. Retrieved from http://www.asha.org/policy

American Speech-Language-Hearing Association. (2008). *Roles and responsibilities of speech-language pathologists in early intervention* [Guidelines]. Retrieved from http://www.asha.org/policy

Arick, J., Krug, D., Fullerton, A., Loos, L., & Falco, R. (2005). School-based programs. In F. Volkmar, R. Paul, A. Klin, & D. Cohen (Eds.), *Handbook of autism and pervasive developmental disorders, Volume Two: Assessment, interventions and policy* (3rd ed., pp. 1103–1028). Hoboken, NJ: Wiley.

Ayers, A. J. (1979). *Sensory integration and the child.* Los Angeles, CA: Western Psychological Services.

Bellini, S. (2006). *Building social relationships: A systematic approach to teach social interaction skills to children and adolescents with autism spectrum disorders and other social difficulties.* Overland Park, KS: Autism Asperger Publishing.

Buron, K. D., & Curtis, M. B. (2012). *The incredible 5-point scale: The significantly improved and expanded second edition: Assisting students in understanding social interactions and controlling their emotional responses.* Overland Park, KS: Autism Asperger Publishing.

Carpenter, M., & Tomasello, M. (2000). Joint attention, cultural learning, and language acquisition: Implications for children with autism. In A. Wetherby & B. Prizant (Eds.), *Autism spectrum disorders: A transactional developmental perspective* (Vol. 9, pp. 31–54). Baltimore, MD: Paul H. Brookes.

Cirrin, F., & Penner, S. (1995). Classroom based and consultative service delivery models for language intervention. In S. Warren & J. Reichle (Eds.), *Language intervention: Preschool through the elementary years* (pp. 333–362). Baltimore, MD: Paul H. Brookes.

Common Core State Standards Initiative. (2012). Retrieved from http://www.corestandards.org/assets/application-to-students-with-disabilities.pdf

Dawson, G., & Zanolli, K. (2003). Early intervention and brain plasticity in autism. In G. Bock & J. Goode (Eds.), *Autism: Neural bases and treatment possibilities. Novartis Foundation Symposium 251* (pp. 266–280).

Diehl, S. F. (2003). The SLP's role in collaborative assessment and intervention for children with ASD. *Topics in Language Disorders, 23*(2), 95–115.

Ehren, B. (2002). Speech-language pathologists contributing significantly to the academic success of high school students: A vision for professional growth. *Topics in Language Disorders, 22*(2), 60–80.

Fisher, D., Frey, N., & Sax, C. (1999). *Inclusive elementary schools: Recipes for success.* Colorado Springs, CO: PEAK Parent Center.

Grandin, T. (2005). A personal perspective of autism. In F. Volkmar, R. Paul, A. Klin, & D. Cohen (Eds.), *Handbook of autism and pervasive developmental disorders: Assessment, interventions, and policy* (Vol. 2, pp. 1276–1286). Hoboken, NJ: Wiley.

Grandin, T. (2006). *Thinking in pictures, expanded edition: My life with autism.* New York, NY: Vintage Books.

Hodgden, L. A. (1996). *Visual strategies for improving communication, volume 1: Practical supports for school and home.* Troy, MI: Quirk Roberts.

Hodgden, L. A. (1999). *Solving behavior problems in autism: Improving communication with visual strategies.* Troy, MI: Quirk Roberts.

Janzen, J. E., & Zenko, C. B. (2012). *Understanding the nature of autism: A guidebook to the autism spectrum disorders* (3rd ed.). San Antonio, TX: Hammill Institute on Disabilities.

Klin, A., Saulnier, C., Tsatsanis, K., & Volkmar, F. (2005). Clinical evaluation in autism spectrum disorders: Psychological assessment within a transdisciplinary framework. In F. Volkmar, R. Paul, A. Klin, & D. Cohen (Eds.), *Handbook of autism and pervasive developmental disorders: Assessment, interventions, and policy* (Vol. 2). Hoboken, NJ: Wiley.

Klinger, L., & Dawson, G. (1992). Facilitating early social and communicative development in children with autism. In S. Warren & J. Reichle (Eds.), *Causes and effects in communication and language intervention* (pp. 157–186). Baltimore, MD: Paul Brookes.

Kranowitz, C. S. (2005). *The out-of-sync child: Recognizing and coping with sensory processing disorders.* New York, NY: Penguin Group.

Landry, R., & Bryson, S. E. (2004). Impaired disengagement of attention in young children with autism. *Journal of Child Psychology and Psychiatry, 45*(6), 1115–1122.

Mahoney, G., & Wiggers, B. (2007). The role of parents in early intervention: Implications for social work. *Children and Schools, 29,* 7–15.

McGee, G. G., Morrier, M. J., & Daly, T. (1999). An incidental teaching approach to early intervention for toddlers with autism. *Research and Practice for Persons with Severe Disabilities, 24* (3), 133–146.

Mundy, P., & Burnette, C. (2005). Joint attention and neurodevelopmental models of autism. In F. R. Volkmar, R. Paul, A. Klin, & D. Cohen (Eds.), *Handbook of autism and pervasive developmental disorders, Vol. 1: Diagnosis, development, neurobiology, and behavior* (3rd ed., pp. 650–681). Hoboken, NJ: Wiley.

Mundy, P., & Neal, A. R. (2001). Neural plasticity, joint attention, and a transactional social-orienting model of autism. In L. M. Glidden (Ed.), *International review of research in mental retardation: Autism* (Vol. 23, pp. 139–168). San Diego, CA: Academic Press.

National Association of Special Education Teachers. (2012). *Examples of IEP goals and objectives: Suggestions for students with autism. Autism Spectrum Disorder Series.* Retrieved from http://www.naset.org/fileadmin/user_upload/Autism_Series/Examples _IEP_Goals_Objectives_for_ASD.pdf

National Autism Center. (2009). *National standards report: The national standards project—Addressing the need for evidence-based practice guidelines for autism spectrum disorders.* Randolph, MA: National Autism Center.

National Research Council. (2001). *Educating children with autism.* Washington, DC: National Academy Press, Committee on Educational Interventions for Children with Autism, Division of Behavioral and Social Sciences and Education.

Neitzel, J., & Wolery, M. (2009). *Implementation checklist for least-to-most prompts.* Chapel Hill, NC: The National Professional Development Center on Autism Spectrum Disorders, FPG Child Development Institute, the University of North Carolina. Retrieved from http://autismpdc.fpg.unc.edu/content/prompting

Prizant, B. M., Wetherby, A. M., Rubin, E., Laurent, A. C., & Rydell, P. J. (2006). *The SCERTS® model: A comprehensive educational approach for children with autism spectrum disorders.* Baltimore, MD: Paul Brookes.

Quill, K. A. (2000). *Do-Watch-Listen-Say.* Baltimore, MD: Paul H. Brookes.

Rao, P., Beidel, D., & Murray, M. (2008). Social skills interventions for children with Asperger syndrome or high functioning autism: A review and recommendations. *Journal of Autism and Developmental Disorders, 38,* 353–361.

Stiles, J. (2000). Neural plasticity and cognitive development. *Developmental Neuropsychology, 18*(2), 237–272.

Stokes, S. (2001). ASD iceberg (handouts from presentation in June 2012 @ CARD). *How do I reference?*

Sussman, F. (1999). *More than words: A guide to helping parents promote communication and social skills in children with autism spectrum disorder.* Toronto, Canada: The Hanen Centre.

Vismara, L. A., Colombi, C., & Rogers, S. J. (2009). Can one hour per week of therapy lead to lasting changes in young children with autism? *Autism, 13,* 93–115.

Vygotsky, L. S. (1978). *Mind in society: The development of higher psychological processes.* Cambridge, MA: Harvard University Press.

Wetherby, A., & Prizant, B. (1989). The expression of communicative intent: Assessment issues. *Seminars in Speech and Language, 10,* 77–91.

Williams, M. S., & Shellenberger, S. (1996). *"How does your engine run?": A leader's guide to The Alert Program for self-regulation.* Albuquerque, NM: Therapy Works.

Winner, M. G., & Crooke, P. J. (2011, January 18). Social communication strategies for adolescents with autism. *ASHA Leader.*

Wolfberg, P. J. (2009). *Play and imagination in children with autism* (2nd ed.). Columbia, NY: Teachers College Press.

5

Interpersonal Communication

Introduction

This chapter focuses on communication between two or more people and how ASD affects this type of interpersonal communication. Understanding how ASD affects each individual's learning styles and behavior is necessary before implementing any communication strategies. Remembering the typical strengths and weaknesses of children on the autism spectrum will help the SLP develop meaningful and effective intervention plans to improve interpersonal communication. In order to cover the broad range of communication abilities demonstrated by children on the autism spectrum, this chapter starts from the emerging communicators and their unique communication challenges and moves all the way through the highly verbal individuals who struggle more with the pragmatic use of language.

According to Merriam-Webster's online dictionary, communication is a process by which information is exchanged between individuals through a common system of symbols, signs, or behavior. As discussed previously in Chapter 3 on assessment, SLPs often divide the language needed to communicate into three main categories: form, content, and use (Bloom & Lahey, 1978). Form is how a message is conveyed (gestures, sign language, words, pictures, Augmentative and Alternative Communication [AAC] device), and what the message looks like in terms of morphology, syntax, and phonology. Content refers to the actual meaning of the message or the semantics. Use refers to pragmatic language or how the form and content are used to communicate in a socially appropriate way (Bloom & Lahey, 1978).

Another way SLPs define communication is in terms of communicative acts and functions. As discussed in Chapter 3 on assessment, communicative functions occur across three main areas: behavior regulation, social interaction, and joint attention (Bruner,

1981). Communicative functions progress from meeting basic wants and needs to communicating in order to share and relate to others socially. These definitions are referenced throughout this chapter to address the needs of children on the autism spectrum at various communicative stages.

The SLP's Role as a Social Communication Interpreter

When the term interpreter is used in the SLP community, it usually refers to someone who relays messages via sign language between a person who is deaf or hard of hearing and the hearing world. However, children and adults on the autism spectrum often need a social communication interpreter who can relay messages to them in a way they understand and then back to the people in the *neurotypical* world (Janzen & Zenko, 2012).

> Neurotypical is a word that was first used by people with autism and Asperger syndrome to describe people who are not on the autism spectrum.

Individuals on the autism spectrum often have difficulty understanding spoken communication and unspoken social cues effectively (Myles, Schelvan, & Trautman, 2004). Therefore, becoming an interpreter who helps translate the complicated and obscure social and verbal language needed to fit in and succeed in the neurotypical world to individuals who are not natural-born social communicators is a pivotal part of the SLP's role.

Interpreters relay messages back and forth, in this case, between individuals on the spectrum and the people in their support network. As a clinician who understands the complex communication process and how the characteristics of ASD affect learning and communication, this makes the SLP uniquely qualified to formulate and translate meaningful messages and successful intervention tools. The more "fluent" the SLP becomes in reading and understanding children with ASD's perspectives, the better the interpreter he or she will be.

A social communication interpreter has to translate both spoken and unspoken messages to the child with ASD, so the world makes more sense. With the sensory processing differences and the social language barrier often present in children with autism, the world often feels like a scary place. Part of the responsibility as a social communication interpreter is to teach families, educators, peers, and other professionals how they can be effective translators to reduce anxiety of the foreign or misunderstood messages. Therefore, the more people who can act as social communication interpreters, translating both social and spoken messages when they occur, the more context-rich opportunities are created for the child with ASD to learn and practice social communication skills successfully.

Emerging Communicators

For the purpose of this chapter, the term *emerging communicator* refers to children who are not using words yet to communicate and just beginning to understand that they can interact with another person to help them get what they want. The SCERTS model refers to this group of children as *Social Partners* (Prizant, Wetherby, Rubin, Laurent, & Rydell, 2006). The SCERTS model is referenced several times throughout this text. To clarify, the authors realize that the SCERTS model is not the only framework out there. However, the basic foundation of meeting the child with autism's sensory and emotional regulation (ER) needs prior to engaging in any type of intervention or instruction of key social communication goals (SC) follows the authors' professional philosophies and the theory of optimal stress for learning outlined in Chapter 2.

To discuss how to improve communication skills of emerging communicators, we need to look back at how early social communication milestones set the stage for the development of spoken language. Infants start socially interacting with the people in their world from birth. At around three to four months of age, *typically developing* infants start to show reciprocal emotional turn-taking (Bates, 1979; Stern, 1985). When caregivers coo, talk, and smile at them, they smile, coo, and giggle back. This continues and as the social communication connection strengthens, the infants begin to initiate the social interactions, babbling, cooing, and smiling before the adult does (Bates, O'Connell, & Shore, 1987; Stern, 1985). By around nine months, infants are able to follow a caregiver's point and gaze and jointly attend to an object or event (Bates, 1979; Prizant et al., 2006). The ability to follow an adult's point, look at the common object or event, and then look back at the caregiver is the definition of joint attention (Bates, 1979). As joint attention develops, the infant not only follows the point or gaze of the adult but starts to initiate this triadic interaction to share enjoyment and focus with the adult (Carpenter & Tomasello, 2000; Cunningham, 2012). This complex social dance happens seamlessly in typically developing infants and sets the stage for the development of verbal communication (Carpenter, Nagell, & Tomasello, 1998; Greenspan, Wieder, & Simons, 1998). The foundation of communication is solidified as the infant engages more and more with caregivers and understands that two people can share enjoyment, comment, and bond over the same item or event (Carpenter et al., 1998). As the natural development of first words comes in to play (around 12 to 14 months), the joint attention episodes are augmented by words and utterances that enhance the interaction and blossom into simple conversations (Bates, 1979; Bloom, 1993; Carpenter et al., 1998; Carpenter & Tomasello, 2000; Mundy & Stella, 2000).

As discussed in previous chapters, one of the earliest, most predictive signs of ASD is the lack of or delay in the development of joint attention (Mundy & Stella, 2000). Typically developing infants' brains are prewired to focus on the social stimuli in their environment (Dawson, Meltzoff, Osterling, Rinaldi, & Brown, 1998; Dawson, Toth, Abbott, Osterling, Munson, Estes, & Liaw, 2004). In contrast, infants who are at-risk and are later diagnosed with ASD have brains that are wired to focus more on the objects in their environment, not the social stimuli (Dawson et al., 1998; Dawson et al., 2004; Mundy

& Neal, 2001). Dawson et al. (1998) coined this failure to naturally orient to the social stimuli in the environment as a *social orientation impairment*. As a result of this social orientation impairment, the early building blocks of communication starting with reciprocal emotional interactions around three to four months old are missing or less frequent, thus creating a gap in the communication development foundation (Dawson et al., 1998; Dawson et al., 2004; Greenspan et al., 1998; Mundy & Neal, 2001; Prizant et al., 2006; Stern, 1985). This creates a domino effect in reverse where the typically developing child's communication tiles start to fall into place, and the child with ASD's dominos are still lined up, not moving.

By the time the child with ASD comes to see a SLP, human nature has often compensated and the child has figured out a way to communicate his or her basic wants and needs. However, these compensatory strategies are not always ideal and are often in the form of challenging behaviors (Fox, Dunlap, & Buschbacher, 2000). Therefore, understanding how the communication foundation may be adversely affected by the way the child with ASD processes social stimuli in the environment is critical for the SLP to recognize so he or she can go back and target some of the missing pieces to strengthen the social communication foundation (Mundy & Neal, 2001).

Where to Start?

For the young child with ASD who shows little interest in others, the biggest goal is to show him or her that people can be fun, interesting, useful, and reinforcing. Sussman (1999) refers to these children being in the *own-agenda* phase; they are only interested in what makes them happy and do not notice others around them. The goal of the clinician for *own-agenda* children (also known as, early communicators or social partners) is to show the child, by creatively manipulating the environment, that the other people in their world hold the key to desired objects, activities, and fun. A few ways to create communication opportunities or temptations include: putting highly desired objects in view but out of reach, offering choices, doing the unexpected, being "the keeper" of desired objects, and doing things wrong on purpose (Sussman, 1999; Wetherby & Prizant, 1989).

For the best results, the clinician should model the strategies for the caregivers, so they can see how to engage their child in a fun, reinforcing way while promoting communication. This helps build the early social communication bonds that did not develop on their own and shows the child the value and fun that the social communication partners can offer (Carpenter & Tomasello, 2000; Mundy & Stella, 2000). By teaching the parents to successfully engage with their children and promote social communication growth by being their social communication interpreter, the clinician has now exponentially increased the opportunities and naturalistic contexts for the child to practice and master the new skills (Koegel, Schreibman, Britten, Burke & O'Neill, 1982; National Research Council, 2001; Stahmer & Gist, 2001; Vismara, Colombi & Rogers, 2009). The clinician has also empowered the parents to feel like they are a part of the solution to help their child gain skills they did not have before and to feel successful as a parent (Brookman-Frazee, 2004; Koegel et al., 1982; Ozonoff & Cathcart, 1998; Vismara et al., 2009). Once the social communication relationship begins to form and develop, a more solid foundation is put in place for receptive and expressive language to grow.

Some resources that are geared to help with building interaction with emerging communicators include: The Hanen Centre's *More Than Words* program (Sussman, 1999), *Relationship Development Intervention with Young Children* (Gutstein & Sheely, 2002), SCERTS (Prizant et al., 2006), *Do-Watch-Listen-Say* (Quill, 2000), and The FirstWords Project (http:// firstwords.fsu.edu). These books and programs focus on building social reciprocity and communication in children on the spectrum. Because ASD is such a broad spectrum, there is not one perfect curriculum or resource that will work for all children. The resources listed above provide a cadre of information and suggestions to pull from when trying to design a meaningful intervention plan.

Form, Content, and Use

In order to discuss the elements needed for a quality treatment plan that addresses expressive, receptive, and pragmatic language goals, this chapter utilizes the form/content/ use definition of communication (Bloom & Lahey, 1978) to outline key interpersonal communication components for each developmental language stage. The goal of any SLP working with a family of an *emerging communicator* is to build opportunities for quality interactions and create an effective, universally understood way for the child to express their wants and needs. The SLP also needs to ensure that the caregivers, family members, teachers, and so forth are able to express their messages in a format or language that is easily understood by the child with ASD.

For emerging communicators, the form of communication is often a combination of vocalizations, signs, gestures, and pictures (Prizant et al., 2006). The main goal is for the child to have a way to use their language in whatever form that works to get their messages across and to understand messages being sent. If a child is using signs, gestures, and pictures to communicate their messages, the caregivers and other people in the support network need to use the same form of language (signs, gestures, and pictures) when trying to communicate with the child with ASD (Burkhart, 2010). This is called Naturally Aided Language (NAL; Van Tatenhove, 2007). Utilizing NAL allows the child to see a model of how to use the form(s) of communication we are trying to teach them to use when the communication partners use the same form(s) to *talk* to them (Burkhart, 2010; Van Tatenhove, 2007).

Once the form(s) of communication has been established, deciding what vocabulary or content to teach is the next task. There are several factors involved when choosing which key vocabulary or semantic concepts to introduce. First, the SLP needs to review what the initial assessment revealed regarding expressive and receptive vocabulary. Next, looking at resources that detail typically developing vocabulary in same-age peers helps provide a framework for selecting age-appropriate content. Utilizing the research from the AAC field on choosing *core vocabulary* words to set up AAC devices is another resource to review when creating intervention plans that identify developmentally appropriate and meaningful expressive and receptive vocabulary words (Pruett, 2011).

> For a comprehensive review of typical language development and how it corresponds to choosing core vocabulary words see:
>
> http://www.vantatenhove.com/files/NLDAAC.pdf
>
> http://www.ttacnews.vcu.edu/2011/05/core-vocabulary-makes-communication-meaningful.html

Key language content will depend on each child's unique environment, interests, and culture. The vocabulary chosen needs to fit the environmental demands for each child, respect cultural differences, and utilize special interest areas for motivation. For example, if the child with ASD is highly motivated by *Thomas the Tank Engine* and is using pictures as their communicative form, the content of several of the pictures may include Thomas-related objects, characters, and so forth.

Finally, teaching a child with ASD to use the language form and content in a socially appropriate manner is the last piece of the communication puzzle. Knowing how to use language in a meaningful and acceptable way is called pragmatics or pragmatic language (Bloom & Lahey, 1978). Communicative functions are at the root of pragmatic language explaining why we communicate. The most basic communicative functions include requesting, protesting, and gaining attention (Bruner, 1981; Wetherby & Prizant, 2002). If a child does not have an effective way to request a desired object or action, protest or refuse an undesired object or action or gain the attention of people around them, they often develop *undesirable* behaviors to convey these basic communicative messages (Fox et al., 2000). As each child begins to develop social or communication skills, the complexity of their communicative functions increase. This is illustrated by the shift of the child's communicative acts from functions that are directed to change other people's behavior, to more social/conversational functions such as commenting, sharing of emotion, and maintaining relationships through social routines (e.g., greetings, turn-taking; Bruner, 1981; Quill, 2000; Shumway & Wetherby, 2009). This shift to more social functions to communicate appears in later communication stages. Finally, as the child begins to understand that communicating allows them to control their environment and create relationships with others, the social communication foundation has added a layer of cement, filling in some of the gaps and providing a more solid base for future learning. Quality intervention plans address all three components of language (form, content, and use) simultaneously because successful communication requires the seamless integration of all three parts of language.

Play and Peer Interaction

As discussed in Chapters 1 and 3, the development of play and communication parallel each other (Bates et al., 1987; McCune-Nicolich & Caroll, 1981). In addition, play has two separate but corresponding continuums of development; the symbolic and social aspects of play (Wolfberg, 2009). During the initial assessment, it is imperative to assess the child's play skills to discover where they are on the play development continuums, so the SLP can see how the child's play skills correlate to their interpersonal communication skills. Therapy involving young children needs to be play-based in order to follow EBP and be meaningful to the child (National Research Council, 2001; Quill, 2000; Wolfberg, 2009). According to Wolfberg (1999), "play is critical to the child's capacity to understand and relate to the social world . . . providing opportunities for children with autism to become competent in play is of prime importance" (p. 5). Therefore, knowing where the child is on both the symbolic and social play skills continuums will help the clinician plan developmentally appropriate intervention.

> See Figures 3–2 and 3–3: Two Dimensions of Play Development in Chapter 3.

If a child has not developed a solid symbol system to communicate, odds are he or she has not developed symbolic play skills. Therefore, creating play scenarios for emerging communicators during therapy should use toys that fall into the sensorimotor and functional categories.

Getting an emerging communicator to interact with another person during a session may be difficult because he or she is developmentally in the solitary stage of the social play continuum. Therefore, gathering information from caregivers regarding the child's favorite type of sensorimotor and functional toys or games is crucial to try and engage the child during therapy. (See the Play Interest Inventory in Quill, 2000). Once you know what toys and games are highly motivating, utilizing the strategies mentioned early in the chapter (be the keeper of the toy, put things in view but out of reach, etc.) will help create natural communicative temptations that focus on gaining the child's attention and thus building language (Carpenter & Tomasello, 2000; Sussman,1999; Wetherby & Prizant, 1989). Modeling this type of child-directed play during therapy will help caregivers see how to foster language development in fun play settings at home. Meeting the child at his or her communication and play levels helps intervention start on a positive note and builds the bridges necessary to bring the child closer to the next communication stage.

Early Communicators

Early communicators are children who have developed some symbolic language and understand that communication involves at least two people, but their language is mostly one- to two-word phrases or simple sentences and utilizes a limited array of communicative functions (Prizant et al., 2006). For the purpose of this chapter, the term early communicators is synonymous with the Language Partner stage from the SCERTS model. Regardless of the term used with this group of children, the primary social communication goals revolve around increasing the amount of words and word combinations used spontaneously in a variety of settings with multiple people. Another main focus of intervention is to develop complex, joint attention skills that promote more social and less behaviorally driven communicative functions (Prizant et al., 2006).

Where to Start?

Always start by reviewing the information gathered during assessment and how ASD affects the child. Next, actively plan how to bring in different people and a variety of settings to implement social communication goals. As stated above, one of the primary goals of this group is to increase the depth of the social interactions by developing their joint attention skills and increasing the amount of words, phrases, and simple sentences. Creating environments with natural opportunities to communicate with different people on a more social (e.g., greeting), less behavioral (e.g., requesting to get something) level is key. The ultimate goal is to have the child with ASD realize that communicating with others on a purely social level can be reinforcing and enjoyable.

The same resources and strategies discussed in the Emerging Communicator section fit for this group of children. Building up expressive and receptive vocabulary is an additional facet of intervention at this stage. Another focus of intervention is broadening the communicative functions beyond the primary ones that control other people's behavior. Utilizing the children's interests is an easy way to help motivate and captivate children on the spectrum's attention thus allowing you to expand their current vocabulary and pragmatic language skills.

> See the accompanying DVD (A–9a and b) for an example of a child being taught about "who" questions using his interest areas.

Form, Content, and Use

The form of communication for early communicators is typically simple one- or two-word phrases and simple sentences. During this stage of communication development, the child is transitioning from using gestures and vocalizations to their first real words and word combinations (Prizant et al., 2006). Knowing that children on the autism spectrum may have difficulty with verbal output, the form of communication during this stage can be spoken words, signed words, picture cards, or any combination of the above (Prizant et al., 2006).

The goal of most families seeking intervention is to have their child speak to communicate. Although speaking is the most efficient and effective way for people to communicate, some children with ASD have a co-occurring motor-speech disorder, like apraxia (Dzuik et al., 2007; Ming, Brimacombe, & Wagner, 2007). If the child has a coexisting motor-speech disorder or is unable to use speech to communicate, the SLP needs to explore augmentative or alternative communication (AAC) options that work for the child. Utilizing various forms of AAC (sign language, picture cards, Voice Output Communication Devices, or Speech Generating Devices) allows the SLP to continue to foster the language development regardless of the speech output difficulties (Beukelman & Mirenda, 2012; Ganz et al., 2012; Mirenda, 2001, 2003). Families are often under the wrong impression that if you use any form of AAC, it will hinder the development of spoken language. On the contrary, research has shown that for children with Childhood Apraxia of Speech, or children with ASD who have trouble using speech to communicate, that continuing to target language development goals using AAC increases the likelihood that speech will develop, if physically possible, and fosters the development of overall communication and language skills (Beukelman & Mirenda, 2012; Cumley, 2001; Cumley & Swanson, 1999; Ganz et al., 2012; Mirenda, 2001, 2003; Rupp, 2013).

Finding the right AAC system for any child is a complex process. The intervention team must consider several factors and allow the child to try various AAC options before making an informed decision on which AAC system to pursue (Beukelman & Mirenda, 2012; Zabala, 2005). Zabala (2005) created the SETT Framework as a guide to help teams map out AAC options that best fit each child or individual. SETT stands for Student Environment Task and Tools. This framework emphasizes the need for the entire team to collaborate and evaluate the individual student's needs that match their environments and give them access to the tasks required for the child to learn and succeed. After the team gathers the student, environment, and task information, then a discussion about what tool(s) or devices would work best for the student follows before making a final decision (Zabala, 2005).

> For more information on AAC assessment, intervention, and best practices go to
> http://www.wati.org
> http://natri.uky.edu/assoc_projects/qiat/about.html
> http://www.aacinstitute.org; or
> http://www.joyzabala.com/Home.php

The Picture Exchange Communication System (PECS; Frost & Bondy, 2002) is one AAC system that is often introduced to the early communicator, at least the first and second phases (Flippin, Reszka, & Watson, 2010). PECS has six phases that reflect the complexity of language as the phase increases. The first phase is focused on teaching the child *how* to communicate using a picture card. The goal of phase I is to teach the exchange of communication. In Phase I, the student is taught to exchange a picture with an adult (with the help of another adult to guide them to be successful in the exchange), and then the adult gives the child whatever is on the picture (Frost & Bondy, 2002).

Phase II focuses on learning to discriminate the pictures that are printed on the card (Frost & Bondy, 2002). The best way to teach the child to discriminate between the pictures is to have a picture of a highly preferred item and a picture of a nonpreferred or neutral item. When the child exchanges the picture with the adult, the adult gives the child whatever is on the card. If the child hands the adult the nonpreferred card and gets the nonpreferred item, some form of protest usually follows. In the moment of protest, the adult shapes the child's response to pick the card of the preferred item, drawing attention to the picture and matching object and then gives the child the desired object. With repetition and practice, the child learns to look at the pictures on the card and make a choice based on the object they want. For a more in-depth explanation of PECS and how to use it with children on the spectrum, see the PECS manual and the meta-analysis of the research published about PECS and ASD (Flippin et al., 2010; Frost & Bondy, 2002).

The content or semantics appropriate for the early communicators goes back to what we know about typical language development. First words usually develop between 12 to 18 months and word combinations around 19 months (Bates, 1979; Bloom, 1993; Prizant et al., 2006; Stern, 1985). Depending on the assessment results of the child's expressive and receptive vocabulary and the developmental norms, the semantic content or words chosen to target should fall between where the child is and where his or her same-age peers are. As always, the content should also reflect meaningful words in the individual's environment, culture, and interests. For early communicators, the SLP should utilize language expansion techniques, using the child's existing expressive vocabulary to build the child's length of spontaneous utterances. For example, if the child points to a picture of a bird in a book and says, "bird," the SLP would expand on the child's expression saying and pointing to the same picture, "blue bird" or "I see the bird. He's in the tree."

The use of language or pragmatics is a focal point of intervention for early communicators. This group understands the basic concept of communicating to get their needs met. Deepening the child's reciprocal communication by expanding their joint attention skills is paramount during this phase. Reciprocal communication is an intricate process that involves sharing attention, sharing affect, and sharing intentions (Prizant et al., 2006).

Communicative intention and communicative functions are not synonymous (Prizant et al., 2006). Intention is what the child wants to happen by communicating. For example, if a child points to a DVD case of his or her favorite movie and says "Nemo," the child's intention is for the adult to grab the Nemo movie and turn it on (request an object-behavior regulation category). If the adult understands the child's intention, he or she will get the movie and turn it on. The function of the child's point and spoken request is fulfilled. However, if the adult looks at the DVD case and responds, "Oh, I love Nemo. That's my favorite movie" without getting the movie down, the adult misread the child's intention and function (request) and followed up with a comment (joint attention category), which does not match the function of the child's intention.

Teaching and understanding communicative functions that regulate people's behavior (requesting, protesting) are much easier and the focus of intervention for emerging communicators. Early communicators need to learn how to communicate to gain someone's attention, the next step on the communicative function ladder, and move towards the last rung of communicating to just to share information about a joint focus (Bruner, 1981; Wetherby & Prizant, 2002). Teaching these last two categories of communicative functions is more difficult given the social delays associated with autism and the social nature of the reinforcement from gaining someone's attention and sharing information (Shumway & Wetherby, 2009; Wetherby & Prizant, 2002).

Children on the autism spectrum do not automatically pick up the social cues surrounding interpersonal communication. Therefore, SLPs need to directly teach joint attention skills like how to secure someone's attention before speaking. Using modeling and role playing are two ways the SLP can teach securing someone's attention by calling their name or tapping them on the shoulder. Greeting people, asking permission, and commenting are three more skills that fall under the more sophisticated joint attention communicative functions and are appropriate for the early communicators (Carpenter & Tomasello, 2000; Prizant et al., 2006; Shumway & Wetherby, 2009).

In addition to role playing and modeling, using video modeling and Social Stories (Gray, 2010) are two other tools shown to effectively teach social skills (National Autism Center, 2009). Recording the children practicing greeting or asking permission and then going back to review it, is a way to use visual strategies that include the children's interest (seeing themselves on film). Social Stories (Gray, 2010) are stories that are written for an individual to help explain social situations in a story format. It is important to match the reading or language level of the story with the developmental level of the child. For example, a Social Story for an early communicator learning about greeting might say:

> I can say hi and bye to my teacher. When I see Ms. Cathy I can say hi. Ms. Cathy will say hi to me too. It makes Cathy happy when I say hi to her. When it is time to go home I can tell Ms. Cathy bye. Ms. Cathy will tell me bye, and she might even wave. I will try to say hi and bye to Ms. Cathy.

The Social Story should include pictures (preferably actual photographs of the child and the teacher) to illustrate each main point. The story is read to the child as a way to teach, prime, and/or review the skill.

Shared book reading is one way to teach, model, and elicit comments in a naturalistic setting. Ideally, the child can pick a book that interests him or her and the illustrations that are already in the book provide perfect visual cues for eliciting commenting. Teaching these more socially-based communicative functions needs to be fun and engineered so the positive rewards that occur after doing the above tasks can reinforce the new functions. More complex communicative functions help foster more complex symbol use and vice versa (Prizant et al., 2006; Shumway & Wetherby, 2009).

Play and Peer Interaction

Early communicators already understand how, albeit on a rudimentary level, to interact with people and can do so with words, phrases, and short sentences, demonstrating they have basic symbolic representation (Prizant et al., 2006). From a play development standpoint, early communicators should be playing with sensorimotor and construction toys and emerging into symbolic play (Wolfberg, 2009). Socially, early communicators should be moving from solitary play into parallel play and emerging into cooperative play with supports (Prizant et al., 2006; Wolfberg, 2009).

Helping an early communicator generalize their communication abilities to different settings with a variety of people is another focus of intervention (Prizant et al., 2006).

Utilizing peers is one way to provide social communication opportunities with different communication partners (Janney & Snell, 2006). Matching peers with similar interests along with toys that are motivating and commensurate with the child's play development stage are necessary for success (Bellini, 2006; Quill, 2000; Wolfberg, 2009). For instance, if the child with ASD likes to build with blocks, try and find peers who are patient, are good language models, and also like to build. The children may need some adult facilitation to keep the interaction going and be productive, but the more child-led the peer interactions can be, the better (Quill, 2000; Wolfberg, 2009).

Engineering play situations with the above recommendations helps provide positive play interactions that are filled with organic language-learning opportunities. Quill (2000) noted "children use play to experiment with their growing knowledge of the world and people" (p. 10). Children with autism often need the guidance of their peers and adult facilitators to get the full benefit of play and its rich communication and learning potential.

Conversational Communicators

This last stage of communication development involves children with autism who have a plethora of expressive language and use all of the communicative functions but struggle most with the social rules or pragmatic part of language. These are the children who often talk in long monologues about their special interest areas, who can answer high-level academic questions, but who struggle with how to join a group of peers and fit in. The more subtle cognitive characteristics like difficulty with executive function, perspective taking (or theory of mind), and central coherence (discussed in Chapter 1) play a pivotal role in designing effective intervention (Baron-Cohen, 2000; Baron-Cohen, Leslie, & Frith, 1985; Happé, 1997; Joseph & Tager-Flusberg, 2004; McEvoy, Rogers, & Pennington, 1993; Ozonoff & McEvoy, 1994; Ozonoff, Pennington, & Rogers, 1991). Difficulty with executive function, perspective taking, and central coherence has a profound effect on social communicative competence. Therefore, it is imperative that the SLP understands how each area of cognitive difficulties affect social communication.

Where to Start?

It is well documented that children on the autism spectrum have difficulty picking up on the nonverbal social cues that envelope all communication exchanges (Attwood, 1998; Myles et al., 2004; Myles & Southwick, 1999; National Research Council, 2001; Rogers, 2000; Winner & Crooke, 2011). In 1971, Mehrabian published a formula he created based on his research of communicative messages. His formula states that the meaning of any spoken communication message is mostly conveyed (93%) by nonverbal cues like body language and tone of voice. More specifically, 7% of any spoken message is conveyed by the actual words spoken; 38% is conveyed by tone of voice, and 55% is conveyed by body language (Mehrabian, 1971). Children with autism who have trouble recognizing the nonverbal cues and who process language literally are left to rely on the actual words being spoken (only 7% of the message meaning) to understand any given communication exchange. These staggering statistics shed a light on where intervention for the conversational communicators needs to begin; start teaching the social skills and social thinking required to interpret nonverbal messages (Mehrabian, 1971; Winner & Crooke, 2011).

There are several resources that provide examples of how and what social or pragmatic skills to teach: *Building Social Relationships* (Bellini, 2006), *Do-Watch-Listen-Say* (Quill, 2000), *Talkability* (Sussman, 2006), *Navigating the Social World* (McAfee, 2002), and *Social Skills Training* (Baker, 2003). Michelle Garcia Winner has several resources listed on her website: http://www.socialthinking.com. Social Thinking teaches children how to think socially by addressing the underlying cognitive difficulties. Three of Winner's books that provide overviews of Social Thinking include: *Inside Out: What Makes a Person with Social Cognitive Deficits Tick?* (2000), *Thinking About You Thinking About Me* (2007), and *Think Social: A Social Thinking Curriculum for School-Age Students* (2008). All of these resources are filled with ideas to create meaningful, socially-driven intervention goals.

Form, Content, and Use

Language form is not usually the main focus of therapy for this group of children on the spectrum. However, continuing to expand the existing language form is best practice. For this group, working on form may include targeting any morphology or syntax concerns. Intervention may also focus on form if there are any articulation or speech sound, stuttering, or voice concerns while targeting the more salient challenges of content and use.

The content to target will vary with each child on the spectrum. One area of semantic language that is especially difficult for children with ASD is figurative or nonliteral language (Happé, 1995, 1997; MacKay & Shaw, 2004). Children on the spectrum interpret language literally; however, the English language is full of figurative language (Happé, 1995). Therefore, the SLP often needs to teach the meanings of idioms, similes, metaphors, humor, and sarcasm using concrete, visual strategies and direct instruction (Janzen & Zenko, 2012; Nippold, 1991).

> The following websites provide fun, visual ways to teach figurative language:
>
> http://www.idiomsbykids.com
>
> http://www.grammarmancomic.com/comics/idioms.html
>
> http://www.idiomsite.com/
>
> http://www.funbrain.com/idioms/
>
> http://www.buzzle.com/articles/metaphor-examples-for-students.html

> The child presented in Case Study B in Chapter 7 is working on figurative and idiomatic language. See B–5 and B–7 on the accompanying DVD.

Understanding the meaning of words is complex and requires the child with ASD to grasp the fundamental concepts most children learn innately. Namely, everyone and everything has a name or label; things can have multiple labels (garbage/trash); and words can have multiple meanings (can, a helper verb; a noun, a cylindrical object; verb meaning to fire, etc.; Janzen & Zenko, 2012, p. 38). Solidifying these semantic concepts helps make communicative exchanges more successful and improve academic performance when these confusing language concepts are understood.

Pragmatic language is the primary focus of interpersonal communication intervention for conversational communicators. Learning the nuances of social rules is crucial for individuals on the spectrum to be socially accepted by their peers, but often the most difficult thing for them to learn (Myles et al., 2004; Winner, 2000, 2007, 2008). In addition, it is often hard for the adults to understand how a person with so much verbal language and intelligence does not understand basic social perspective taking, such as that it is rude to tell someone they are fat, even if by definition they are. The person with autism may just be telling the truth because when they were young, they were taught the rule, "do not lie." Children on the spectrum do not pick up on the unspoken rule that at a certain point, people expect you to tell "white lies" to avoid hurting another person's feelings (Myles et al., 2004). The literal nature of their brains holds on to the rule that says not to lie, so they tell the truth.

Difficulty with perspective taking or theory of mind is at the root of several of the pragmatic difficulties of the conversational communicators (Baron-Cohen, 2000; Baron-Cohen et al., 1985; Winner, 2000, 2007, 2008). In order to build social relationships with others, a basic knowledge of human emotions, how to read them in others, and how your behavior may effect their emotions is required (Baron-Cohen, 2000; Baron-Cohen et al., 1985). Resources like the Social Thinking products aim to teach children and adults on the spectrum how to read emotions, see others' perspectives, and alter their behavior according to how their social partners are feeling. The SLP working with conversational communicators needs to teach basic perspective taking, reading emotions, and hidden social rules in a concrete manner. For a comprehensive list of resources that target teaching social skills, see Winner (2007, pp. B4–B5).

> Case Studies B and C provide examples of children working on skills within the conversational communicator phase. The DVD provides multiple examples of materials used with these children to teach the hidden rules about conversation and building and maintaining relationships (Case Study B: B–3, B–8; Case Study C: C–1, C–2, and C–6).

Play and Peer Interaction

Conversational communicators have the language and the symbolic representation to participate in symbolic play and interact with other children, with supports (Prizant et al., 2006). Depending on the age of the child, utilizing play in therapy may or may not be appropriate. For older children, using integrated social groups that target social communication goals is common (Bellini, 2006; Winner, 2000, 2007). Integrating the use of peer-models to teach and learn social skills for conversational communicators is essential (Bellini, 2006; Janney & Snell, 2006). Peers need to be briefed on what to expect, what ASD is, and how they can act as mentors and friends. Once the peers are given the information and instructions, they typically jump right in and the age-appropriate social interactions begin (Bellini, 2006; Janney & Snell, 2006; Quill, 2000). Peer-mediated intervention has proved to be effective for teaching children on the autism spectrum (National Autism Center, 2009; National Research Council, 2001)

Utilizing visual strategies like Comic Strip Conversations (Gray, 1994), Social Stories (Gray, 2010), and Social Autopsies (Bieber, 1994) work for children on the autism spectrum (National Research Council, 2001). The common denominator of all the above strategies is using visual techniques to illustrate abstract social situations in a concrete format. Children on the spectrum can be taught social skills, but often need the SLPs to help them literally connect the dots between what happened and why. Therefore, utilizing visual strategies helps create a visible map for the children to follow, explaining how the social and communication worlds relate (Gray, 1994, 2010; Janzen & Zenko, 2012).

Video modeling is another strategy shown to effectively teach social skills (Bellini, 2006; Bellini & Akullian, 2007; National Autism Center, 2009). Utilizing existing videos of TV shows, movies, or on YouTube and pausing them to illustrate the social goal is one way of using video modeling. Vargin (2012) outlines how to use videos with additional visual supports (like Post-It notes on the screen) to concretely dissect social situations and teach appropriate skills. Video self-modeling involves recording the student doing a desired task, with adult prompts if necessary, and then editing out the prompts (Bellini & Akullian, 2007). Once the prompts are removed from the video, the clinician shows the child the footage of him or herself doing the desired skill successfully and independently. The combination of the dynamic visual model of the child watching him or herself complete the targeted skill independently and successfully has shown positive outcomes (Bellini, 2006; Bellini & Akullian, 2007; National Autism Center, 2009).

Finally, Myles et al. (2004) outline ways to teach children on the spectrum about the *Hidden Curriculum*. Their book helps identify what the hidden curriculum items are for children of various ages and provide suggestions how to teach each concept. Myles (2011, personal communication) shared a story of how one school used the hidden curriculum daily calendar (Myles & Duncan, 2008) on the morning news. The principal would read the hidden curriculum goal of the day, and then the entire school would practice using the appropriate skills. Reading a daily hidden curriculum item originally started to help a few students with autism in the school, but the teachers reported that most of their students benefitted from the daily reminder of appropriate social behavior.

Summary

Interpersonal communication skills require all three parts of language to be successful. Promoting the development of social communication is one of the primary roles of SLPs working with children on the autism spectrum. Intervention goals vary for each child depending on where he or she is on the communication continuum. For *emerging communicators* or the more preverbal children, fostering interaction and joint attention are at the heart of language intervention. For *early communicators* who are starting to use a few words and short phrases, continuing to foster the joint attention and interaction is still critical. Adding more emphasis on building and expanding the semantic and pragmatic areas of language is recommended. Finally, for the highly verbal, *conversational communicators*, major emphasis is placed on improving the pragmatic use of language to build social competence and peer relationships. There are several strategies outlined in this chapter to help improve the interpersonal communication skills of children throughout the autism spectrum. All of the strategies follow the balanced intervention pyramid premise of taking into account the learning strategies common in ASD, using assessment data to know where to start and then utilizing interventions that are proven to work with this population.

Learning Tool

1. Name one key area of interpersonal communication intervention for a child in the emerging communicator, early communicator, and conversational communicator phase.

2. Why is perspective taking important to interpersonal communication?

3. Describe the two continuums of play development and how they relate to communication development.

References

Attwood, T. (1998). *Asperger's syndrome: A guide for parents and professionals.* Philadelphia, PA: Jessica Kingsley.

Baker, J. E. (2003). *Social skills training: For children and adolescents with Asperger syndrome and social-communication problems.* Shawnee Mission, KS: Autism Asperger Publishing.

Baron-Cohen, S. (2000). Theory of mind and autism: A fifteen year review. In S. Baron-Cohen, H. Tager–Flusberg, & D. J. Cohen (Eds.), *Understanding other minds: Perspectives from developmental cognitive neuroscience* (pp. 3–20). Oxford, UK: Oxford University Press.

Baron-Cohen, S., Leslie, A. M., & Frith, U. (1985). Does the autistic child have a "theory of mind"? *Cognition, 21,* 37–46.

Bates, E. (1979). *The emergence of symbols: Cognition and communication in infancy.* San Diego, CA: Academic Press.

Bates, E., O'Connell, B., & Shore, C. (1987). Language and communication in infancy.

In J. Osofsky (Ed.), *Handbook of infant development* (pp. 149–203). New York, NY: Wiley.

Bellini, S. (2006). *Building social relationships: A systematic approach to teaching social interaction skills to children and adolescents with autism spectrum disorders and other social difficulties.* Shawnee Mission, KS: Autism Asperger Publishing.

Bellini, S., & Akullian, J. (2007). A meta-analysis of video modeling and video self-modeling interventions for children and adolescents with autism spectrum disorders. *Exceptional Children, 73*(3), 264–287.

Beukelman, D., & Mirenda, P. (2012). *Augmentative and alternative communication: Supporting children and adults with complex communication needs* (4th ed.). Baltimore, MD: Paul H. Brookes.

Bieber, J. (1994). *Learning disabilities and social skills with Richard LaVoie: Last one picked . . . first one picked on* [DVD]. Washington, DC: Public Broadcasting Service.

Bloom, L. (1993). *The transition from infancy to language.* New York, NY: Cambridge University Press.

Bloom, L., & Lahey, M. (1978). *Language development and language disorders.* New York, NY: Wiley.

Brookman-Frazee, L. (2004). Using parent/clinician partnerships in parent education programs for children with autism. *Journal of Positive Behavior Interventions, 6,* 195–213.

Bruner, J. (1981). The social context of language acquisition. *Language and Communication, 1,* 155–178.

Burkhart, L. (2010). Aided language stimulation: Research to practice. Retrieved from http://www.lburkhart.com/ATIA_ALgS_handout_1_10.pdf

Carpenter, M., Nagell, K., & Tomasello, M. (1998). Social cognition, joint attention, and communicative competence from 9 to 15 months of age. *Monographs of the Society for Research in Child Development, 63*(4, Serial No. 255), 1–143.

Carpenter, M., & Tomasello, M. (2000). Joint attention, cultural learning, and language acquisition: Implications for children with autism. In A. Wetherby & B. Prizant (Eds.), *Autism spectrum disorders: A transactional developmental perspective* (Vol. 9, pp. 31–54). Baltimore, MD: Paul H. Brookes.

Cumley, G. D. (2001). *Children with apraxia and the use of augmentative and alternative communication.* The Childhood Apraxia of Speech Association of North America. Retrieved from http://www.apraxia-kids.org/library/children-with-apraxia-and-the-use-of-augmenative-and-alternative-communication/

Cumley, G. D., & Swanson, S. (1999). Augmentative and alternative communication options for children with developmental apraxia of speech: Three case studies. *Augmentative and Alternative Communication, 15*(2), 110–125.

Cunningham, A. B. (2012). Measuring change in social interaction skills of young children with autism. *Journal of Autism Development and Disorders, 42,* 593–605.

Dawson, G., Meltzoff, A., Osterling, J., Rinaldi, J., & Brown, E. (1998). Children with autism fail to orient to naturally occurring social stimuli. *Journal of Autism and Developmental Disorders, 28,* 479–485.

Dawson, G., Toth, K., Abbott, R., Osterling, J., Munson, J., Estes, A., & Liaw, J. (2004). Early social attention impairments in autism: Social orienting, joint attention, and attention to distress. *Developmental Psychology, 40*(2), 271–283.

Dzuik, M. A., Gidley Larson, J. C., Apostu, A. A., Mahone, E. M., Denckla, M. B., & Mostofsky, S. H. (2007). Dypraxia in autism: Association with motor, social and communicative deficits. *Developmental Medicine and Child Neurology, 49,* 734–739.

Flippin, M., Reszka, S., & Watson, L. R. (2010). Effectiveness of the picture exchange communication system (PECS) on communication and speech for children with autism spectrum disorders: A meta-analysis. *American Journal of Speech-Language Pathology, 19,* 178–195.

Fox, L., Dunlap, G., & Buschbacher, P. (2000). Understanding and intervening with children's problem behavior: A comprehensive approach. In S. F. Warren & J. Reichle (Series Eds.) and A. M. Wetherby & B. M. Prizant (Vol. Eds.), *Communication and language intervention series: Vol. 9. Autism spectrum disorders:*

A transactional developmental perspective (pp. 307–331). Baltimore, MD: Paul H. Brookes.

Frost, L., & Bondy, A. (2002). *Picture exchange communication system (PECS) training manual.* Newark, DE: Pyramid Educational Consultants.

Ganz, J. B., Earles-Vollrath, T. L., Heath, A. K., Parker, R. I., Rispoli, M. J., & Duran, J. B. (2012). A meta-analysis of single case research studies on aided augmentative and alternative communication systems with individuals with autism spectrum disorders. *Journal of Autism and Developmental Disorders, 42,* 60–74.

Gray, C. (1994). *Comic strip conversations: Colorful illustrated interactions with student with autism and related disabilities.* Jennison, MI: Jennison Public Schools.

Gray, C. (2010). *The new social story book, revised and expanded 10th anniversary edition: Over 150 social stories that teach everyday social skills to children with autism or Asperger's syndrome, and their peers.* Arlington, TX: Future Horizons.

Greenspan, S. I., Wieder, S., & Simons, R. (1998). *The child with special needs: Encouraging intellectual and emotional growth.* Reading; MA: Addison-Wesley.

Gutstein, S. E., & Sheely, R. K. (2002). *Relationship development intervention with young children: Social and emotional development activities for Asperger syndrome, autism, PDD, and NLD.* London, England: Jessica Kingsley.

Happe, F. G. C. (1995). Understanding minds and metaphors: Insights from the study of figurative language in autism. *Metaphor and Symbolic Activity, 10,* 275–295.

Happé, F. G. E. (1997). Central coherence and theory of mind in autism: Reading homographs in context. *British Journal of Developmental Psychology, 15*(1), 1–12.

Janney, R., & Snell, M. (2006). *Social relationships and peer support, second edition (Teachers' guides to inclusive practices).* Baltimore, MD: Paul H. Brookes.

Janzen, J. E., & Zenko, C. B. (2012). *Understanding the nature of autism: A guidebook to the autism spectrum disorders* (3rd ed.). San Antonio, TX: Hammill Institute on Disabilities.

Joseph, R. M., & Tager-Flusberg, H. (2004). The relationship of theory of mind and executive functions to symptom type and severity in children with autism. *Developmental Psychopathology, 16*(1), 137–155.

Koegel, R. L., Schreibman, L., Britten, K. R., Burke, J. C., & O'Neill, R. E. (1982). A comparison of parent training to direct child treatment. In R. L. Koegel, A. Rincover, & A. L. Egel (Eds.), *Educating and understanding autistic children* (pp. 260–279). San Diego, CA: College-Hill Press.

MacKay, G., & Shaw, A. (2004). A comparative study of figurative language in children with autistic spectrum disorders. *Child Language Teaching and Therapy, 20*(1), 13–32.

McAfee, J. (2002). *Navigating the social world: A curriculum for individuals with Asperger's syndrome, high functioning autism and related disorders.* Arlington, TX: Future Horizons.

McCune-Nicolich, L., & Carroll, S. (1981). Development of symbolic play: Implications for the language specialist. *Topics in Language Disorders, 2,* 1–15.

McEvoy, R. E., Rogers, S. J., & Pennington, B. F. (1993). Executive function and social communication deficits in young autistic children. *Journal of Child Psychology and Psychiatry, 34,* 563–578.

Mehrabian, A. (1971). *Silent messages* (1st ed.). Belmont, CA: Wadsworth.

Ming, X., Brimacombe, M., & Wagner, G. (2007). Prevalence of motor impairment in autism spectrum disorders. *Brain and Development, 29,* 565–570.

Mirenda, P. (2001). Autism, augmentative communication and assistive technology: What do we really know? *Focus on Autism and Other Developmental Disabilities, 16*(3), 141–151.

Mirenda, P. (2003). Towards functional augmentative and alternative communication for students with autism: Manual signs, graphic symbols, and voice output communication aids. *Language, Speech, and Hearing Services in Schools, 34,* 203–216.

Mundy, P., & Neal, R. (2001). Neural plasticity, joint attention and a transactional social-orienting model of autism. In L. Glidden (Ed.), *International review of research in mental retardation. Autism* (Vol. 23, pp. 139–168). New York, NY: Academic Press.

Mundy, P., & Stella, J. (2000). Joint attention, social orienting and communication in autism. In S. F. Warren & J. Reichle (Series Eds.) and

A. M. Wetherby & B. M. Prizant (Vol. Eds.), *Communication and language intervention series: Vol. 9. Autism spectrum disorders: A transactional developmental perspective* (pp. 55–77). Baltimore, MD: Paul H. Brookes.

Myles, B. S., & Duncan, M. (2008). *2009 hidden curriculum one-a-day calendar*. Shawnee Mission, KS: Autism Asperger Publishing.

Myles, B. S., Schelvan, R., & Trautman, M. L. (2004). *The hidden curriculum: Practical solutions for understanding unstated rules in social situations*. Shawnee Mission, KS: Autism Asperger Publishing.

Myles, B. S., & Southwick, J. (1999). *Asperger Syndrome and difficult moments: Practical solutions for tantrums, rage and meltdowns*. Shawnee Mission, KS: Autism Asperger Publishing.

National Autism Center. (2009). *National standards report: The national standards project—Addressing the need for evidence-based practice guidelines for autism spectrum disorders*. Randolph, MA: National Autism Center.

National Research Council. (2001). *Educating children with autism*. Washington, DC: National Academy Press, Committee on Educational Interventions for Children with Autism, Division of Behavioral and Social Sciences and Education.

Nippold, M. A. (1991). Evaluating and enhancing idiom comprehension in language-disordered students. *Language, Speech, and Hearing Services in Schools, 22*, 100–106.

Ozonoff, S., & Cathcart, K. (1998). Effectiveness of a home program intervention for young children with autism. *Journal of Autism and Developmental Disorders, 28*, 25–32.

Ozonoff, S., & McEvoy, R. E. (1994). A longitudinal study of executive function and theory of mind development in autism. *Development and Psychopathology, 6*, 415–431.

Ozonoff, S., Pennington, B. F., & Rogers, S. J. (1991). Executive function deficits in high-functioning autistic individuals: Relationship to theory of mind. *Journal of Child Psychology and Psychiatry, 32*, 1081–1105.

Prizant, B. M., Wetherby, A. M., Rubin, E., Laurent, A. C., & Rydell, P. J. (2006). *The SCERTS model: A comprehensive educational approach for children with autism spectrum disorders*. Baltimore, MD: Paul Brookes.

Pruett, M. D. (2011). *Core vocabulary makes communication meaningful*. Retrieved from http://www.ttacnews.vcu.edu/2011/05/core-vocabulary-makes-communication-meaningful.html

Quill, K. A. (2000). *Do-watch-listen-say*. Baltimore, MD: Paul H. Brookes.

Rogers, S. (2000). Interventions that facilitate socialization in children with autism. *Journal of Autism and Developmental Disorders, 30*, 399–330.

Rupp, D. F. (2013). *Augmentative and alternative communication (AAC) for children with apraxia*. The Childhood Apraxia of Speech Association of North America. Retrieved from http://www.apraxia-kids.org/library/augmentative-and-alternative-communication-aac-for-children-with-apraxia/

Shumway, S., & Wetherby, A. M. (2009). Communicative acts of children with autism spectrum disorders in the second year of life. *Journal of Speech, Language, and Hearing Research, 52*, 1139–1156.

Stahmer, A. C., & Gist, K. (2001). The effects of an accelerated parent education program on technique mastery and child outcome. *Journal of Positive Behavior Interventions, 3*, 75–82.

Stern, D. (1985). *The interpersonal world of the infant*. New York, NY: Basic Books.

Sussman, F. (1999). *More than words: A guide to helping parents promote communication and social skills in children with autism spectrum disorder*. Toronto, Canada: The Hanen Centre.

Sussman, F. (2006). *TalkAbility: People skills for verbal children on the autism spectrum: A guide for parents*. Toronto, Canada: The Hanen Centre.

Van Tatenhove, G. (2007). *Normal language development, generative language & AAC*. Retrieved from http://www.vantatenhove.com/index.html

Vargin, A. (2012). *Movie time social learning*. San Jose, CA: Think Social Publishing.

Vismara, L. A., Colombi, C., & Rogers, S. J. (2009). Can one hour per week of therapy lead to lasting changes in young children with autism? *Autism, 13*(1), 93–115.

Wetherby, A., & Prizant, B. (1989). The expression of communicative intent: Assessment issues. *Seminars in Speech and Language, 10*, 77–91.

Wetherby, A. M., & Prizant, B. (2002). *Communication and symbolic behavior scales developmental profile—First normed edition.* Baltimore, MD: Paul Brookes.

Winner, M. G. (2000). *Inside out: What makes a person with social cognitive deficits tick?* San Jose, CA: Think Social Publishing.

Winner, M. G. (2007). *Thinking about YOU thinking about ME* (2nd ed.). San Jose, CA: Think Social Publishing.

Winner, M. G. (2008). *Think social! A social thinking curriculum for school-age students* (2nd Printing). San Jose, CA: Think Social Publishing.

Winner, M. G., & Crooke, P. J. (2011, January 18). Social communication strategies for adolescents with autism. *ASHA Leader.*

Wolfberg, P. J. (2009). *Play and imagination in children with autism* (2nd ed.). Columbia, NY: Teachers College Press.

Zabala, J. S. (2005). *Using the SETT framework to level the learning field for students with disabilities.* Retrieved from http://www.joyzabala.com/uploads/Zabala_SETT_Leveling_the_Learning_Field.pdf

6

Communication
for Learning

Introduction

This chapter reviews communication and language skills needed to succeed in an academic setting. Integrating how the characteristics of ASD, especially the unique cognitive differences in perspective taking, executive function, and central coherence, affect all areas of learning is highlighted throughout the various academic domains. Strategies that help improve academic learning and communication based on the underlying cognitive characteristics of ASD and how the SLP fits into the educational process is presented.

Children with ASD have been noted to have lower academic achievement than predicted based on their intellectual ability (Estes, Rivera, Bryan, Cali, & Dawson, 2011). As outlined in Chapter 1, individuals with ASD often have difficulty with perspective taking, executive function, and central coherence (Baron-Cohen, 1989; Baron-Cohen, Leslie, & Frith, 1985; Frith, 1989; Happé, 1997; Myles & Southwick, 1999). These cognitive differences and core difficulties with social and communication skills have a major impact on learning and academic success (Estes et al., 2011; Jones et al., 2009; Norbury & Nation, 2011). The SLP serves an important role to help the child with ASD improve social communication skills and access the learning environment.

> See Chapter 3 on assessment for more information on the characteristics of social communication in children with ASD

Executive functions include several cognitive operations, including: working memory, inhibition, mental flexibility, and planning (Joseph & Tager-Flusberg, 2004; McEvoy,

Rogers, & Pennington, 1993; Ozonoff & McEvoy, 1994; Ozonoff, Pennington, & Rogers, 1991). An aspect of executive function that frequently appears to be impaired in children with ASD is attention (Ciesielski, Courchesne & Elmasian, 1990; Courchesne, 1991; Frith & Baron-Cohen, 1987; Quill, 1997). More specifically, Courchesne (1991) found impairments in the rapid shifting of attention; Ciesielski et al. (1990) found delays in shifting attention between visual and auditory stimuli; and Frith and Baron-Cohen (1987) found impairments in attending to the most meaningful feature of a stimulus. This is consistent with many teacher and parent reports of attention difficulties observed at home and/or in the classroom.

When you think of how a typical classroom environment is set up, students are expected to attend to a myriad of auditory and visual input, make judgments regarding what is the most important stimuli at any given moment, and then integrate all the incoming information in a meaningful way. In addition to the attentional demands and decisions, the students have to simultaneously comprehend the verbal and nonverbal communication from the teacher and other students and derive the correct meaning from all of this information. For children with ASD who have difficulty with perspective taking, executive function (including shifting attention and paying attention to multiple stimuli) and central coherence (seeing the "big picture"), learning in a typical classroom is often challenging without the proper supports. Therefore, the SLP is often asked to expand their role as a social communication interpreter for children on the spectrum (discussed in Chapter 5) to include interpreting the academic or instructional demands. For the SLP in an educational setting, this expanded role may be structured within the Response to Intervention (RTI) process. Justice (2006b) outlines important ways the SLP can be involved with the RTI process within all tiers, including providing consultative support to the general education teams providing Tier 1 instruction, assisting with the design of interventions and instructional approaches, and helping to monitor progress. Utilizing the knowledge of how the unique characteristics of ASD affect the learning style of children with autism will help the SLP translate the classroom demands and instructional discourse into a format that children with ASD can understand.

Instructional Discourse

Instructional or classroom discourse is the language used in an instructional setting between the teacher(s) and students (Nutall, Graesser, & Person, 2013). The typical classroom discourse pattern involves the teacher lecturing or doing a presentation, asking a question, a student or students respond, and the teacher comments or provides feedback on the student(s)' answers (Nutall et al., 2013). Lectures are often followed up with individual seatwork that students complete independently (Applebee, Langer, Nystrand, & Gamoran, 2003). This pattern is referred to as I-R-E (initiation, response, evaluation) and relies mostly on verbal communication (Applebee et al., 2003).

Quill (1997) provides an overview of the early research that shows that children with ASD learn better with visual cues that augment the primarily verbal classroom environments (Hermelin & O'Connor, 1970; MacDuff, Krantz, & McClannahan, 1993; Quill & Grant, 1996; Schopler, Mesibov, & Hearsey, 1995). Therefore, one of the first steps an SLP working with a child in a school setting can do is go observe the child in the classroom and discover what the classroom discourse style entails. If the learning environment reflects the more verbal, I-R-E model, creating visual supports to help the student with ASD take in instructional information that makes sense to him or her and have a way to respond is critical. This is when the SLP becomes the academic or instructional interpreter for the child on the spectrum. Modeling how to use a more visual teaching style that utilizes visual supports often helps ensure the teacher will accept and use the supports created. When the visual supports help improve the academic outcomes of the student(s) with ASD in a faster, more efficient way, the other students often ask if they can use the supports. A simple example is creating a visual schedule that the student with ASD can use to guide him or her through an academic routine (Figure 6–1).

Another helpful strategy for students with ASD is a color-coded word problem key that identifies specific words that signal the student to use one of the four main mathematical operations (addition, subtraction, multiplication, division). Matching the color-coded blocks for each operation with a corresponding highlighter gives the student a way to visually mark the *operation* words in the word problem to help him or her focus on the necessary math calculations to solve the problem (Figure 6–2).

Providing visual cues often helps decrease the presence of challenging behaviors in the classroom because the student(s) on the spectrum are less anxious and more successful when the information they are expected to learn makes sense. Following is one example of how the visual learners with autism may feel in a primarily verbal-based instructional model.

> *Imagine yourself taking a calculus course for the first time. All of the material is new to you, difficult to grasp, and your teacher is from a foreign country and speaks with a heavy foreign accent. He is speaking English, the language you should understand, but you have to concentrate so hard to understand what he is saying that it is twice as hard to get the calculus lesson's key points. Most of your cortical energy is being used up trying to decipher the words your teacher is saying; therefore, comprehending the difficult new concept is almost impossible. This is how children with ASD often feel on any given school day. They know the language, but they are trying so hard to understand what is being said with all the distractions and "foreign" nonverbal language. If your calculus professor would just write on the board, step by step, the universal language of numbers would help bridge the language barrier. This is why visual supports are so important.*

Visual cues for students with ASD are like the subtitles in a foreign movie. The visuals provide the information in a language they understand. With the challenges students on the spectrum have with perspective taking and reading other people's emotions, they often have difficulty gauging how they are doing or self-monitoring their progress. Because children with ASD cannot automatically sense if they are having a *good day* or a *bad day*,

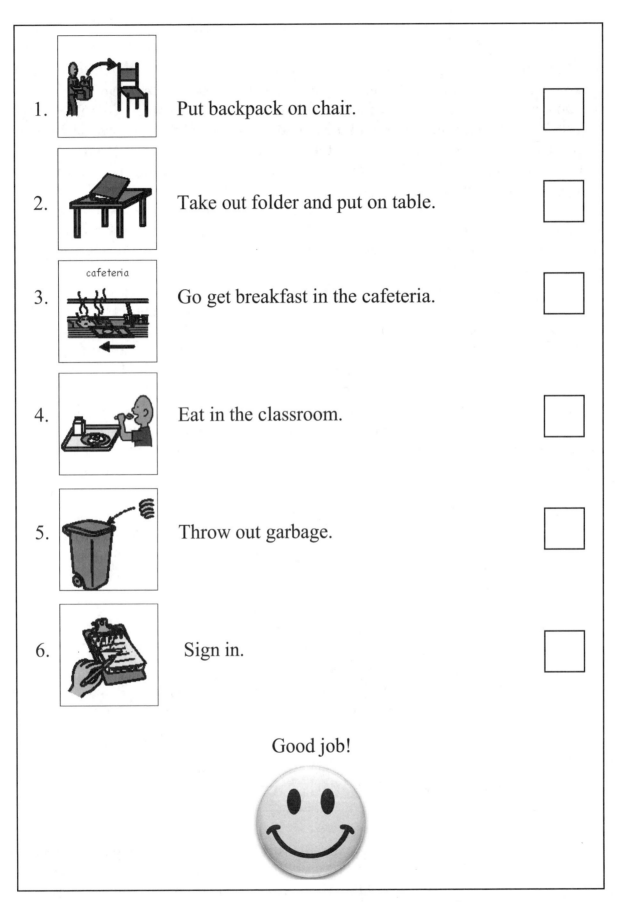

1. Put backpack on chair. ☐

2. Take out folder and put on table. ☐

3. Go get breakfast in the cafeteria. ☐

4. Eat in the classroom. ☐

5. Throw out garbage. ☐

6. Sign in. ☐

Good job!

Figure 6–1. Visual schedule example—create with BoardMaker® software.

ADDITION WORDS (+)	SUBTRACTION WORDS (-)	MULTIPLICATION WORDS (×)	DIVISION WORDS (÷)
All together Sum In all More	Fewer Less than Minus Take away	Product	Quotient

Figure 6–2. Math vocabulary chart—Students can add words to the chart as they encounter them in word problems.

this requires understanding what behavior and actions equal a good or bad rating. Teaching children on the spectrum how to measure their success or answer the question, "How was your day?" is important. Sometimes, the language delays impede students with autism's ability to verbally report back to parents or caregivers how their day was, so the SLP can help develop a visual support to help the child answer the above question.

See Case Study A–1 through A–3 on the DVD for examples.

Ideally, creating an independent and successful student who can coexist in a classroom setting and learn is the goal of most educational teams. Self-monitoring skills are part of the above equation. Therefore, the SLP may need to help create concrete visual markers (for example, smiley faces, stars, check marks, etc.) that are given to show the concepts "that's it" or "needs improvement," so the student can see how he or she is doing throughout the day. Being able to self-monitor and adjust their behavior accordingly is a significant step for students with ASD to be a successful member of their class.

Literacy Development in Children with ASD

Westby (2002) noted that "literacy is an extension of language learning to print" (p. 73). As previously discussed, children with ASD present with difficulties in the area of social communication that can be associated with a wide range of deficits across any of the linguistic components (i.e., semantics, syntax, morphology, phonology, and/or pragmatics), as well as the core cognitive characteristics associated with ASD. It has been well-established in research that children with language disorders in general are at greater risk for literacy disorders (Catts, Fey, Zhang, & Tomblin, 1999; Catts & Kamhi, 1999). The linguistic difficulties that children with ASD face contribute to their increased risk for experiencing challenges with developing literacy skills (Jones et al., 2009; Lanter, Watson, Erickson, & Freeman, 2012; Nation, Clarke, Wright, & Williams, 2006; Norbury & Nation, 2011). Nevertheless, children with ASD *can* develop literacy skills and learn to use these skills meaningfully (Mirenda, 2003; Mirenda & Erickson, 2000).

> See Chapter 3 on assessment for more information on the characteristics of social communication in children with ASD.

Several aspects of cognitive and linguistic function have been linked to the difficulties with literacy development experienced by children with ASD. Research has shown that children's oral language is positively correlated with their literacy levels (Jones et al., 2009; Lanter et al., 2012; Nation et al., 2006; Norbury & Nation, 2011). In a study by Norbury and Nation (2011), children with ASD were found to have difficulty with reading comprehension that was attributable to both oral language skills and to cognitive characteristics associated with ASD. The authors speculated that central coherence difficulties could be at the root of the difficulty that many children with ASD have with getting the overall meaning (global coherence) rather than solely specific details (local coherence; Norbury & Nation, 2011). Additionally, executive function skills, such as being able to suppress irrelevant information or to shift attentional focus (e.g., switching from the specific detail focus to big picture main ideas), may negatively affect performance on comprehension of text (Norbury & Nation, 2011; O'Connor & Klein, 2004). Similarly, Jones et al. (2009) noted that reading comprehension difficulties were not just associated with oral language difficulties, but with the children's social and communication impairments as measured by the ADOS. Figure 6–3 illustrates the relationships between key cognitive and linguistic aspects and how these relate to written language development.

Children with ASD present with a variety of difficulties in literacy development (Jones et al., 2009; Norbury & Nation, 2011). Children on the spectrum ranged so widely in literacy skills in a study by Nation et al. (2006), that their performance scores varied all the way from floor to near ceiling across the reading measures administered. It is important to note that there is not one profile of literacy development associated with a diagnosis of ASD (Jones et al., 2009; Norbury & Nation, 2011). Additionally, while the development of the components of reading (word recognition, decoding, reading accuracy, reading comprehension) have been found to be correlated in typically developing children, Nation et al. (2006) noted that "in children with ASD, component reading skills have a tendency to develop out of step with each other" (p. 915).

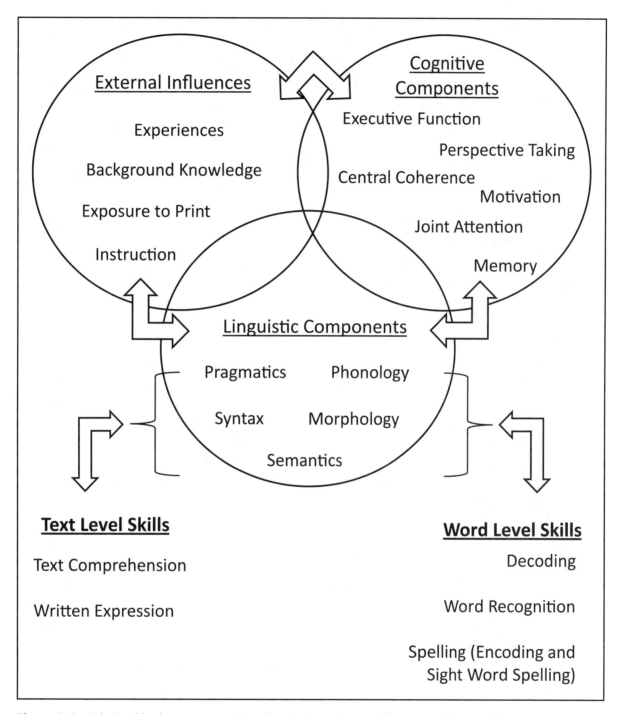

Figure 6–3. Relationships between cognitive, linguistic, and external factors and the core literacy components.

Clinicians must determine the *individual* child's pattern of literacy development before designing an intervention plan. One aspect of reading does stand out as being the most difficult for children with ASD as a group: reading comprehension (Jones et al., 2009; Nation et al., 2006; Norbury & Nation, 2011). This has been linked with deficits in language skills and social communication, as well as to cognitive characteristics associated with ASD (Jones et al., 2009; Norbury & Nation, 2011). As text grows increasingly complex through the school-age years, the difficulty children with ASD face with integration of information (e.g., integrating prior knowledge with information they read) likely negatively affects performance on higher level analysis of text (O'Connor & Klein, 2004).

Even though there is a significant correlation between children with ASD's oral language skills and their literacy development, they are not always predictive of each other in those with ASD. Norbury and Nation (2011) showed "many individuals with significant language impairment could, nevertheless, read single words at an age-appropriate level" (p. 204). In fact, there are individuals with ASD who learn to read and spell without producing spoken language (Mirenda, 2003). Therefore, despite the presence of communication disorders in children with ASD, it is important for the clinician to understand that targeting literacy in intervention should not be withheld until a certain level of oral language has been achieved or they have been judged "ready to read" (Justice, 2006a; Koppenhaver & Erickson, 2003; Mirenda, 2003). There have been some reports in the literature that written language assists with the development of spoken language for some children with ASD (Koppenhaver & Erickson, 2003; Mirenda, 2003). Written communication has the benefit of temporal permanence; the message on the page is not transient like spoken messages and can be taken in at one's own pace or can be reviewed to assist with comprehension (Hodgden, 1999). Perhaps these children develop symbolic language best through literacy, without the *confusing* nonverbal language interference. An excellent example is D. J. Savarese, a young man with autism who learned to communicate through reading and writing. He has written several accounts on how he communicates through writing and how learning to read and write gave him the ability to communicate with people (Savarese, 2010).

Targeting Emergent Literacy in Children with ASD

Although it has not always been a focus of intervention, emergent literacy is an important part of an intervention or educational plan for children with ASD (Lanter et al., 2012). Emergent literacy skills are predictive of later literacy achievement (National Early Literacy Panel, 2008). According to a meta-analysis conducted by the National Early Literacy Panel (2008), the key components that predicted later literacy achievement for all children included:

- Alphabet knowledge
- Phonological awareness
- Rapid automatic naming
- Phonological memory
- Writing, including name writing
- Knowledge of print concepts
- Oral language

As with any aspect of intervention, the clinician should first assess emergent literacy to determine the child's profile of skills. The SLP should be sure to assess across the components of emergent literacy, because children with ASD may show strengths in the "form," such as letter naming/recognition (Lanter et al., 2012), as compared with components rooted in *content* or *use*. In a recent study by Lanter et al. (2012), children with ASD often had difficulty with one or more of the following aspects of emergent literacy:

- Letter-sound correspondence may be less developed than letter naming
- Print concepts (e.g., tracking print left to right, top to bottom; understanding that print has meaning)
- Pretend reading, which is related to difficulties with the print-meaning connection
- Phonological awareness
- Emergent writing, especially for a communicative purpose
- Decreased initiations by the child with ASD for shared book reading.

There has been little attention given to emergent literacy in children with ASD in the research literature (Lanter et al., 2012). The clinician can combine the research specific to children with ASD with what has been learned about evidenced-based practices for emergent literacy instruction for typical or other disordered populations. Justice (2006a) notes that emergent literacy interventions with all children should incorporate a balanced program within the four broad domains of emergent literacy: print knowledge, phonological awareness, writing, and oral language. In the intervention study by Koppenhaver and Erickson (2003), the authors noted that children with severe communication impairments made gains in emergent literacy when provided with many opportunities to explore print in different ways with varying materials (e.g., computer-based access to letter practice, emergent writing practice, many types of paper/pencils/crayons/markers, a wide variety of books that may have appealing sensory components, etc.). The children in the study also benefited from adult-child interactions with various literacy materials and when the children were given time to explore the literacy materials on their own (Koppenhaver & Erickson, 2003). There are specific evidence-based strategies the SLP can utilize within intervention, which are summarized in Table 6–1 (Justice, 2006a; Justice & Pullen, 2003; Koppenhaver & Erickson, 2003; Lanter & Watson, 2008; Zucker, Ward, & Justice, 2009).

Finally, an important part of any intervention program is involving the family and providing education. Lanter et al. (2012) noted that the parents in their study did not demonstrate a complete view of emergent literacy when describing their children's literacy behaviors, often leaving out many critical aspects related to the *content* and *use* of literacy (e.g., understanding the function of print, story comprehension). These parents perceived their children with ASD had a strength in the area of literacy, likely due to their focus on the *form* of literacy, such as letter naming. The SLP can help educate the parents about how to emphasize the meaning and purposes of print, such as encouraging story comprehension and retelling, how to ask higher level analysis questions, providing scaffolds to help the children respond, and how to choose books that contain the right level

Table 6–1. Evidence-Based Strategies for Emergent Literacy Instruction

Instructional Strategy:	Description:
Shared-Book Reading	Adult and child participate in a shared-book reading. Adult may use a variety of techniques to encourage interaction and maximize oral and written language learning (see below).
Dialogic Reading	During shared-book reading, the adult uses specific behaviors that encourage interaction and experience with the text. Includes asking open-ended questions, expanding on children's answers, asking further questions related to the children's comments and questions, giving positive feedback for children's interactions, and following the child's lead and interest areas.
Print Referencing	During shared-book reading, the adult uses techniques to increase the child's awareness of and interest in various aspects of print (e.g., tracking print, asking child to point to where the adult should start reading, asking questions about letters and words on the page, commenting on words, etc.).
Explicit-Embedded Balance	Provide opportunities for the child to be exposed to targeted concepts within natural contexts, but also provide direct instruction.
Literacy-Enriched Play Settings	Embedding literacy props within natural play settings (e.g., having menus and paper/pencil to take someone's order in a restaurant play schema) in order to increase opportunities for emergent literacy exposure in natural, familiar contexts.
Teacher-Directed Structured Phonological Awareness Curricula	Explicit phonological awareness instruction provided through a structured curriculum. Examples of curricula include: *Ladders to Literacy* (Notari-Syverson, O'Connor, & Vadasy, 1998), *Sound Foundations* (Byrne & Fielding-Barnsley, 1991), and *Road to the Code* (Blachman, Ball, Black, & Tangel, 2000).
Mediated Writing	Emergent writing opportunities with adult guiding and scaffolding representation of print concepts.

of complexity to help their child with comprehension and retelling (Lanter et al., 2012). Finally, the SLP can help both parents and teachers increase the opportunities for interaction with literacy materials by collaborating and making sure there are many literacy materials and tools accessible to the child within natural environments (Koppenhaver & Erickson, 2003).

School-Age Literacy Intervention

The SLP's knowledge of how to provide intervention for language deficits is invaluable when designing the educational program for children with ASD. Lanter and Watson (2008) voiced a call to action to SLPs to modify "existing speech-language interventions to include a literacy focus" (p. 33). The common core state standards call for all children to increase understanding of greater text complexity and "improve access to rigorous academic content standards for students with disabilities" (National Governors Association Center for Best Practices, Council of Chief State School Officers, 2010). Language and literacy learning are seen as key building blocks toward achieving successful outcomes in adulthood, as noted in the Report of the National Reading Panel (National Institute of Child Health and Human Development, 2000), which stated that reading comprehension specifically is "essential not only to academic learning in all subject areas but to lifelong learning as well." The SLP can be a key member of the educational team to help determine how students with ASD can meet the expectations of today's academic environment.

Because there is not one profile of literacy development associated with children with ASD, the SLP will need to determine which aspects of literacy require targeting within intervention. Typically the areas of concern in written language parallel those in spoken language. As stated previously, the school-age child with ASD may present with literacy at any level, from learning emergent skills, to "learning to read," all the way up to learning to use complex texts to "read to learn." The available research can give the SLP an idea regarding some general trends of difficult literacy concepts for children with ASD. The following list summarizes component areas of literacy that have been documented to be difficult for *some* children with ASD at some point during the school-age years and may be prime areas to target in intervention (Estes et al., 2011; Jones et al., 2009; Lanter et al., 2012; Nation et al., 2006; Norbury & Nation, 2011; O'Connor & Klein, 2004):

- Emergent literacy learning might be characterized by strength in form (e.g., letter naming) over content (e.g., understanding the function of print)

- Difficulty with phonological awareness; may be in contrast with strengths with letter naming/recognition (Diehl, Ford, & Federico, 2005)

- Difficulty with learning to read words (word recognition and decoding) or spell words; whereas others have a particular strength in this area

- Decreased decoding (nonword reading), even though word recognition skills are within normal limits

- Reduced text level reading accuracy

- Word recognition can become progressively difficult over time, even in children with ASD that have typical *structural* language skills

- Wide range of difficulty with reading comprehension, from difficulty with basic comprehension of text to decreased higher level analysis of text. These difficulties might include:

  ○ Difficulty with comprehension monitoring

  ○ Decreased evaluative skills; including inferencing and prediction skills

  ○ Reduced application of prior knowledge to help interpret text

  ○ Difficulty with anaphoric referencing, or when the text refers back to previous elements within itself using a linguistic signal, particularly with pronouns.

Ultimately, the design of the intervention plan will depend on the specific profile of skills observed during the assessment. The intervention plan might need to be code-focused, meaning-focused, or a combination of both (Whalon, Al Otaiba, & Delano, 2009). See the section above for recommendations for school-age children with ASD who continue to be at the Emergent Level. There is little research available specific to language and literacy intervention of children with ASD. The clinician can combine knowledge regarding the learning styles of children with ASD and established research regarding what types of literacy instruction have been proven effective for children in general. Once again, collaborating with the family and the school professionals is key to developing an intervention plan that addresses the most important targets for successful learning in the classroom.

In keeping with the spirit of this book, children with ASD should be provided balanced literacy instruction (Mirenda, 2003). Balanced literacy means just what the title implies; it is a balance between all of the key features associated with literacy learning: fluency, vocabulary, comprehension, phonics, phonemic awareness, and writing. A balanced literacy approach does not have any prerequisites that a student must master before they are worthy of reading and writing instruction. All students are given equal opportunities to experience the full range of literacy instruction (Cunningham, 1979; Cunningham & Allington, 2010; Cunningham, Hall, & Sigmon, 1999; Erickson & Koppenhaver, 2007).

The Four Blocks Literacy Framework was developed by Cunningham, Hall, and Defee (1991). This framework follows the balanced literacy approach and offers four key areas of literacy instruction on a daily basis: guided reading, self-selected reading, writing, and working with words. Within these four blocks, comprehension, vocabulary, fluency, decoding, and writing composition are all addressed in a fun, meaningful way. The self-selected reading section allows students with ASD to choose and practice reading books about their areas of interest, thus increasing their motivation to read. The writing block allows time for students on the spectrum to write about their interests as well as other topics in a meaningful way. The writing block emphasizes the creative process of writing composition, not handwriting. Often students with ASD need to use alternative pencils (e.g., computer, stand-alone keyboards like the AlphaSmart/Neo2 or Fusion, dictation, dictation software like Dragon Dictate, word-prediction software) to capture their thoughts while avoiding any coexisting fine-motor or motor-planning difficulties (Erickson & Koppenhaver, 2007).

> The following websites have information on stand-alone keyboard systems available:
>
> http://www.writerlearning.com/special-needs/
> http://www.neo-direct.com/default.aspx

The guided reading section helps improve overall language concepts and comprehension skills and opens up an avenue to discuss the characters feelings, actions, and reactions using a concrete, visual reference—the book. Finally, the working with words block helps students understand the patterns of words, sound combinations, and spelling.

Word Level Reading and Spelling

Whereas some children with ASD demonstrate a particular strength in the area of word level reading and spelling skills, many struggle to develop these skills (Norbury & Nation, 2011). Reading and spelling of words are related processes that draw from the same underlying linguistic foundations: phonology, orthography (letters and letter patterns), and morphology (Apel, Masterson, & Hart, 2004; Treiman & Bourassa, 2000). Children with language disorders in general have been noted to be more likely to have difficulty with decoding, word recognition, spelling of familiar words, and/or encoding (Catts & Kamhi, 1999). The SLP's understanding of language, including phonology and morphology, is valuable to help figure out exactly why an individual child is having trouble with word level skills and to develop an intervention plan to remediate the issues. When doing an assessment of reading (decoding and word recognition) and spelling (encoding and sight word spelling), the SLP is encouraged to analyze children's reading miscues and spelling errors according to what level of linguistic breakdown they represent (Silliman, Bahr, & Peters, 2006). The study by Silliman, Bahr, and Peters (2006) describes a method for analyzing the spelling errors based on the underlying linguistic components within the phonological, orthographic, and morphological assessment of spelling (POMAS). Spelling error analysis in particular is an excellent diagnostic tool to help determine which linguistic aspects are difficult for the child and ultimately design an intervention plan to remediate the foundational linguistic skills and specific types of word forms that are difficult for that individual child. For an example of the application of POMAS to various spelling errors see Table 6–2.

Utilizing qualitative analyses of the reading and spelling of progressively complex words will greatly assist the clinician with determining intervention targets. Once these

Table 6–2. Qualitative Analysis of Spelling Errors Using the POMAS Method

| Qualitative Analysis of Spelling Errors Using the POMAS Method | |
| Different misspellings of the word "curls," as in "The girl has curls in her hair." | |
Spelling Error	**Linguistic Component and Feature Misspelled**
Culs	Phonological error; the vocalic "r" sound is not represented.
Kerls	Orthographic error; all sounds and morphemes are represented; the error is on the letters/letter patterns chosen.
Curl	Morphological error; the final regular plural marker has been omitted.
Kul	Phonological, Orthographic, and Morphological errors all present; phonological error: vocalic "r" is omitted; orthographic error: the initial /k/ sound is spelled incorrectly; morphological error: the regular plural marker is not present.

targets have been established, the SLP matches the plan with evidence-based strategies for instruction of difficult patterns.

The following is a list of suggestions for how to target word level reading and spelling skills within intervention. These suggestions are based on existing research about interventions with children with ASD, children with language disorders, and/or best educational practices for children in general.

- Intervention should target decoding and encoding skills in addition to sight word skills, even for those children with ASD with severe communication impairments (Mirenda, 2003; Whalon et al., 2009). Explicit teaching of spelling increases both spelling and reading skills (Berninger, Abbott, Abbott, Graham, & Richards, 2002).

- Target the different linguistic areas in concert (Multiple Linguistic Factor Approach): phonology, morphology, and orthography (Apel, Masterson, & Hart, 2004).

- When working on phonological awareness, connect speech-motor patterns and articulator placement to phoneme perception and manipulation (Troia, 2004).

- Use visuals to make phonological awareness, decoding, and encoding practice more salient (Troia, 2004). Use pictures and place holders (squares, blocks, markers of some sort). It is known that visual supports often increase comprehension and learning for children with ASD. Commonly used visual cues for use during speech sound instruction can be used when working on sound-letter correspondence. For instance, the child could have a picture of a balloon popping that correlates with the /p/ sound.

- Integrate interventions for phonological awareness, letter recognition, and letter-sound training (Troia, 2004). It is important that these skills are not worked on in isolation only, particularly for children with ASD because they are often known to have difficulty with integration of learned information.

- Teach inflectional and derivational morphology, providing instruction about how prefixes and suffixes add additional meaning to root words. Explain that words can be spelled based on letter(s)-sound correspondences, but also based on letter-meaning connections in many multisyllabic words.

- Practice *code-focused* skills (phonological awareness, sound-letter correspondences, letter knowledge, and their application to decoding/encoding) in text rather than just at the word level, so that the children understand these are not just isolated skills (see review by Whalon et al., 2009).

- Utilize a wide range of technologies (Mirenda, 2003). There are many available computer-based programs and applications (apps) to practice word reading and spelling skills. Computer-assisted instruction has been shown in a few studies to be an effective method for decoding and spelling practice (Whalon et al., 2009).

- Provide instruction in use of *multiple strategies* to read or spell words, which might include: sounding out, analogy strategy (using knowledge of familiar words or word families, such as "light" to spell "fright"), sight word strategy, syllabication strategy (dividing words into syllables to read/spell), or morphological strategy (dividing words into roots, prefixes, and suffixes to read/spell and determine word meaning). Calhoon (2001) found that some children with ASD preferred use of an analogy strategy.

Developing Reading Comprehension and Writing Composition Skills

Difficulties with reading comprehension and written expression are frequently observed in children with ASD. At the root of these difficulties is typically a deficit in linguistic skills in semantics, syntax, phonology, morphology, and/or pragmatics. As discussed earlier, the cognitive characteristics associated with ASD also likely negatively affect text comprehension and written expression. See Figure 6–3 for an illustration of these relationships. The SLP is in a unique position to determine which foundational skills should be targeted in intervention. Oral language difficulties often translate to related deficits in text comprehension. For instance, the child who has difficulty with comprehension of complex sentences in spoken language will often experience the same difficulty when reading them. The same child may also have difficulty formulating complex sentence structure, and writing will most likely be composed of simple sentence structures. See the next section for more information on integrating language and literacy intervention.

When addressing reading comprehension skills, it is important for the clinician to choose appropriate texts. Particularly during the early grades, some texts might be designed more for accuracy, word reading practice. If the clinician is looking to target comprehension, then it is important to choose well-structured texts that are within reach of the student's language level (Lanter & Watson, 2008). Children with ASD need to be exposed to a variety of texts, including both narrative and expository structures. Whereas narratives are often regarded by clinicians as being easier for children with language disorders, this might not always be the case for children with ASD (Randi, Newman, & Grigorenko, 2010). Expository texts are factually based with "impersonal, logical" dimensions (Westby, Culatta, Lawrence, & Hall-Kenyon, 2010). Children with ASD often have specific areas of interest and may be particularly motivated to read expository texts surrounding these topics (Lanter & Watson, 2008). Narrative texts require interpretations of problems, identification of solutions, and perspective-taking regarding characters' emotions, beliefs, and intentions; all skills that are often difficult for children with ASD due to underlying cognitive linguistic characteristics (Randi et al., 2010). However, the clinician should be aware that as the child progresses into middle and high school, expository text will become increasingly complex, and these texts may become more difficult for children with ASD due to cognitive and learning characteristics.

Once a text has been chosen, there are strategies that may be helpful to assist students with ASD to expand comprehension skills. As discussed previously, there is little research that looks at effectiveness of particular reading comprehension interventions with children with ASD. First, the clinician can look at which instructional strategies have been found to be evidence-based for children in general. The meta-analyses by the National Reading Panel (National Institute of Child Health and Human Development, 2000) determined which instructional strategies were the most effective for teaching reading comprehension. The following is a list of the seven evidence-based targets and instructional strategies for reading comprehension instruction that were identified:

- Teaching Comprehension Monitoring: Readers actively construct meaning during reading and monitor their understanding while reading.

- Using Graphic and Semantic Organizers: Use of visual supports to assist with comprehension of the material. (See Case Study B–6 on the DVD for video example.)

- Story Structure Instruction: The child is taught the general structure associated with different types of texts (e.g., narratives, expository text, etc.). Knowing the structure has been shown to help children with recalling story information.

- Teaching Summarization: Teaching the children to identify key information and integrate ideas.

- Question Answering: The instructor poses guided questions to help the child reach a deeper meaning of the text. (See Case Study B–2 and B–4 on the DVD for video examples.)

- Question Generation: Children are taught to ask themselves questions about pertinent information from the story.

- Cooperative Learning: Students learn about reading strategies from each other.

It is important to note that the instructional methods listed above are based on research in *typical populations*. The clinician needs to take into account what is known about the learning style, cognitive characteristics, and language skill profile of the individual child with ASD before determining how reading comprehension should be targeted. The following list provides suggestions for strategies to target reading comprehension of children with ASD:

- Use **dialogue** to help the child construct meaning during reading (Lanter & Watson, 2008).

- Use **anaphoric cuing** to help the child keep track of referents, particularly for those with syntactic difficulties (O'Connor & Klein, 2004).

- **Visual-based techniques** may assist with recall of factual information, sequences of information. Visuals used should be instructional supports and paired with "supportive, interactive dialogue" by the clinician (Lanter & Watson, 2008, p. 41). Examples include:
  ○ Mental imagery/visualization,
  ○ Drawing key details in sequence,
  ○ Acting out the story,
  ○ Graphic organizers, including to help demonstrate evaluative concepts, such as cause-effect, compare/contrast (Lanter & Watson, 2008). Graphic organizers

can also be paired with pictures (e.g., semantic web with pictures drawn to represent key details and central idea),

- ○ Comic strip conversations to visually illustrate and teach character perspectives (Gray, 1994).

- Target comprehension and use of **mental state terms**. Sun and Wallach (2013) noted that "mental state terms, including *metacognitive* (realize, understand, imagine, etc.) and *metalinguistic* verbs (explain, argue, agree, etc.), represent people's internal mental states and play important roles in social and conversational understanding" (p. 62). Mental state terms can help cue the reader about internal states of characters.

- **Summarization** in particular has been noted to be especially effective in assisting students' reading comprehension (Westby et al., 2010). Summarizing requires the child to go beyond simply recalling facts, such as in a "retell" (Westby et al., 2010). The child has to integrate information in the text, draw conclusions, make inferences, and glean the overall gist; all aspects that are particularly difficult for the child with ASD due to underlying difficulties with central coherence, perspective-taking/theory of mind, and executive function. Explicitly teach children how to construct a summary, such as: identify important points, review points and remove redundant items or unimportant details, determine how the details are "all the same," and write a main idea sentence. Some word processing programs have summarization tools built in to the application (e.g. Microsoft Word, PC version).

- Target a **deeper understanding** of the text. Provide instruction in how to target higher level analysis, such as inferencing, prediction, perspective-taking (Lanter & Watson, 2008). It is important to remember that many children with ASD may be skilled at recalling specific factual information, yet struggle to integrate information and reach a higher level of comprehension (Lanter & Watson, 2008).

- Provide language experiences to build **background knowledge** before reading as needed (Lanter & Watson, 2008). Multimedia and technology can assist with providing this information in some instances. For example, if discussing or reading about a "parade" and the child has not experienced one, can show a YouTube video of a parade to provide some experience and build background knowledge.

- Prime **prior knowledge** before reading (Lanter & Watson, 2008). However, O'Connor and Klein (2004) found that some students with ASD were distracted by their own tangential or perseverative thoughts, so the clinician needs to help the students actually apply this prior knowledge to text.

- Explicitly teach **types of questions** and how to get the information needed to answer them. Diehl, Ford, and Federico (2005) described an intervention for a child with ASD where they utilized explicit teaching of the four types of questions posed by Raphael (1984): (1) Right There, (2) In My Head, (3) Think and Search, and (4) On My Own. The authors also used visual cues to represent each one.

- Use **multisensory teaching techniques**. The Story Grammar Marker and Braidy the StoryBraid by MindWing Concepts, three-dimensional, tactile story mapping tools, are a form of graphic organizers but provide a tangible object that students can see and touch (see http://www.mindwingconcepts.com/index.htm).

- Encourage the child to **self-identify** which learned strategies he or she might use in given situations. Many children with ASD become used to adults guiding them through problem solving. It is important for them to be an active participant in deciding which strategy to use for given situations (e.g., if working to recall specific details or sequences from text, the child might choose to use visualization or a graphic organizer to note key points). Provide a *strategy bank* where the choices are written down, and the student can select the strategy they want to use.

- Teach **active reading**. Children with ASD need to be continually self-monitoring for comprehension and evidence an active participation in reading. **Self-monitoring** is likely an area of difficulty for children with ASD and several of the recommended strategies by the National Reading Panel in essence encourage this during reading (i.e., text monitoring, question generation, and use of graphic/semantic organizers). Whalon et al. (2009) recommend a self-monitoring checklist to serve as a visual cue for when to stop and ask questions during reading (i.e., question generation strategy). Once the clinician has explained the visual, this visual cue should assist the child with being independent with the cued strategy. Another strategy is to write down the comprehension questions on Post-It notes and have the student place the note in the text while they are reading and come upon an answer.

An important component of language and literacy intervention is written expression. Although clinicians might typically think of "writing" practice as separate from "reading" practice, research reveals important links between the two aspects of literacy. Providing direct instruction for increasing the complexity of writing (i.e., written expression) may help the child develop other related skills. Diehl et al. (2005) found a parallel between one child with ASD's development of narrative and expository text in writing and an increase in language complexity in spoken language. The *Writing to Read: Evidence for How Writing Can Improve Reading* report (Graham & Hebert, 2010) noted writing instruction and intervention can increase reading comprehension. Three specific instructional practices for writing were identified as improving reading:

1. **Have students write about what they read.** This includes summarizing what they read, write responses to material read (requires analysis, interpretation), take notes about what they have read, or answer/create questions about the story.

2. **Explicitly teach writing skills and processes.** For reading comprehension, teach the writing process, macrostructure of different types of text, and paragraph and sentence formulation skills. For reading fluency, target spelling

and sentence construction skills. For word reading skills, explicitly teach spelling skills.

3. **Increase the opportunities students have to write.** Reading comprehension skills can be increased by children having more writing experiences.

4. **Teach the editing process visually.** Utilize the built-in "track changes" mode of most word processing programs. Sometimes children with ASD who interpret language literally will have trouble accepting the concept of writing multiple drafts. In their mind, once they have written the assignment, they are finished. Allowing students to do their first draft on the computer and then use the track changes mode in the same document to show they have gone back through the assignment and made some editorial changes makes the rewrite process less arduous.

Integrated Language and Literacy Intervention

Oral and written language typically develops in parallel. The breakdowns that occur in underlying spoken language are often seen in written language. Synchronizing spoken and written language comprehension goals helps the child make connections between oral and written language. Text may be an effective vehicle for language learning, making language visual and assisting with processing. Children with ASD need to be taught to comprehend the language complexity found in written language, so that it can be accessed for learning.

A great example of pairing oral and written language targets could be targeting comprehension and use of pronouns, especially in increasingly complex sentences. Pronouns have been found to be difficult for children with ASD in both spoken and written language (O'Connor & Klein, 2004; Paul, 2005). It is hard for children with ASD to keep track of what or who the pronouns are referring to within connected text (anaphoric referencing; O'Connor & Klein, 2004). The clinician could work on pronouns in spoken sentences, while in the same session practicing reading sentences and figuring out what the pronouns within paragraphs are referring. Anaphoric cuing while reading text was found to be an effective strategy, such as having students choose the correct referent from a bank of options when encountering pronouns in text (O'Connor & Klein, 2004). This cuing likely reminds the child to monitor comprehension of the text and focuses on an area of difficulty, particularly for those with structural language difficulties. The children can also be asked to formulate sentences in writing and then revise sentences to insert pronoun options presented in word banks. The child with ASD would then be working on the same underlying linguistic concept of comprehension and use of pronouns in: spoken language, reading comprehension, and within writing.

Many of the evidence-based targets for "reading comprehension" are true for intervention aimed at spoken discourse as well. Summarization, question generation, comprehension monitoring, question answering, and anaphoric referencing are all skills important to comprehension of both oral and written discourse. The research supports interventions targeting these skills, and the SLP can help the student with ASD apply the skill in spoken language and when reading and writing text. Many children have difficulty with extending comprehension beyond the basic details stated in text or said in oral discourse. Mental imagery/visualization techniques paired with visual aids to illustrate what the student visualizes can greatly assist these children with learning to inference. For instance, the sentence, "The boy stomped down the hall and threw his books in his locker" evokes images of a boy with an angry facial expression, even though it was not explicitly stated.

There are many skills and strategies the child with ASD can be taught to help with actively listening in the community and in the classroom. This is especially true for comprehension of instructional discourse in the classroom, as it is often primarily verbal in nature (Applebee et al., 2003). Teaching the child to summarize is particularly important. Relatedly, the child can be taught a key word extraction strategy and then learn to paraphrase lengthy text using key words. Once the child has learned to determine key points, learning to find the "main idea," or how these key points are similar, will be much easier. Many children with ASD can be observed to have great difficulty with key word extraction, likely due to their underlying difficulties with central coherence. Intervention can target key word extraction in both text and when listening to instructional or conversational discourse. Students can use highlighters when they are searching and identifying key words in text. Memory strategies may also assist the child with comprehension of discourse, including visual strategies such as mental imagery/visualization. The child could also use visual supports such as semantic maps or mnemonics, or learn to count steps when given complex instructions.

Pragmatic language is a particularly important area to target within both conversation and text for children with ASD. Narratives offer opportunities for the child to explore character perspectives and inference about other people's intentions, and make predictions about what characters might do. These same skills are required in conversational discourse and can be practiced in small group social communication interventions. "Through discussion-based approaches, students have the opportunity to relate their personal experiences, emotions, and feelings to the content and brainstorm potential action plans to solve different interpersonal and social conflicts" (Sun & Wallach, 2013, p. 63). Explicit instruction in the meaning and use of mental state terms can be implemented within conversational discourse, as well as exploring these word types in reading and using the terms in written discourse.

Accommodations and Modifications

Aside from providing direct intervention to the child with ASD, there are supports that can be given by any caregivers and school-based professionals. As previously discussed, the learning style of children with ASD is often mismatched with the way instruction is provided in many classrooms. Often, the child with ASD can participate in general education classrooms when provided supports to accommodate for their learning style and/ or emotional regulation needs. The supports given can include accommodations and/or modifications that can be provided within the classroom during daily instruction and/ or testing situations. There is a big difference between accommodations and modifications. Accommodations are supports that help the child participate in the least restricted learning environment and help them make sense of the language of the classroom. Accommodations support or change *how* the child is instructed or tested. For instance, within the classroom the child may be given written directions on a Post-It note instead of only hearing them verbally. The child might also be given a graphic organizer during reading practice to assist with story comprehension. During testing, the child might be given unlimited time or administered tests in small groups or individually. So the child with accommodations continues to access the same curricular content as the rest of the class, which in terms continues to expose him or her to content that will be covered in annual assessments of progress.

In contrast, modifications change *what* the child is taught. A child with a modification in reading might be taught using a different curriculum that is at their individual reading level. It is important for clinicians to understand the difference between accommodations and modifications, so that the SLP can help figure out which supports best meet the child and family's long-term goals. If the child and family are looking for the child to continue toward graduation with a standard diploma, then accommodations are preferable because the child will continue to be exposed to content needed to pass annual assessments. If the curriculum is modified, the requirements needed to receive a standard diploma are often compromised. All accommodations and modifications should be formally documented. One place accommodations and modifications can be documented is on the child's IEP. Some children with ASD may have a Section 504 plan instead of an IEP, which is a plan for accommodations and/or modifications to be provided to the child with disabilities (Department of Health and Human Services, Office for Civil Rights, 2006). The Section 504 plan in an educational setting does not outline direct interventions provided to the child, rather makes provisions for accommodations or modifications to be made so that the individual can fully access the learning environment.

> See Chapter 4 for more information regarding IEPs.

Summary

The SLP plays an important role in helping children with ASD successfully access the learning environment. When considering the individual profile of cognitive characteristics associated with ASD and the language skills of the child, the SLP can help design an educational or intervention plan and provide direct intervention to improve language skills. The SLP serves as a social communication interpreter and helps the child attain the academic or instructional demands of the classroom. Another important area of instruction that benefits greatly from the expertise of the SLP is literacy development. Children with ASD are significantly at risk for literacy disorders across one or more components (i.e., word recognition, decoding, spelling by sight, encoding, reading comprehension, or writing). SLPs' knowledge of the components of language is a valuable tool for helping to design the intervention or educational plan for children on the spectrum due to the linguistic basis of literacy. Spoken and written language goals can be integrated so that the intervention provided by the SLP helps the child improve communication in both modalities. By working on foundational oral, and written language skills, the SLP can provide skills needed for the child to access content area instruction.

Learning Tool

1. How does the learning style of children with ASD affect their performance in the classroom?

2. How can we help children with ASD understand instructional discourse or the language of the classroom?

3. Name three evidence-based strategies that can be used to increase the reading and writing skills of children with ASD.

4. Write a goal that is designed to target a skill within both spoken and written language.

References

Apel, K., Masterson, J. J., & Hart, P. (2004). Integration of language components in spelling. In E. R. Silliman & L. C. Wilkinson (Eds.), *Language and literacy learning in schools* (pp. 292–318). New York, NY: Guilford Press.

Applebee, A. N., Langer, J. A., Nystrand, M., & Gamoran, A. (2003). Discussion-based approaches to developing understanding: Classroom instruction and student performance in middle and high school English. *American Educational Research Journal, 40*(3), 685–730.

Baron-Cohen, S. (1989). The autistic child's theory of mind: A case of specific developmental delay. *Journal of Child Psychology and Psychiatry, 30*(2), 285–297.

Baron-Cohen, S., Leslie, A. M., & Frith, U. (1985). Does the autistic child have a "theory of mind"? *Cognition, 21*, 37–46.

Berninger, V. W., Abbott, R. D., Abbott, S. P., Graham, S., & Richards, T. (2002). Writing and reading: Connections between language by hand and language by eye. *Journal of Learning Disabilities, 35*, 39–56.

Blachman, B. A., Ball, E. W., Black, R., & Tangel, D. M. (2000). *Road to the code: A phonological awareness program for young children.* Baltimore, MD: Brookes.

Byrne, B., & Fielding-Barnsley, R. (1991). *Sound foundations.* Sydney, New South Wales, Australia: Peter Leyden Educational.

Calhoon, J. A. (2001). Factors affecting the reading of rimes in words and nonwords in beginning readers with cognitive disabilities and typically developing readers: Explorations in similarity and difference in word recognition cue use. *Journal of Autism and Developmental Disorders, 31*, 491–504.

Catts, H. W., Fey, M. E., Zhang, X., & Tomblin, J. B. (1999). Language basis of reading and reading disabilities: Evidence from a longitudinal investigation. *Scientific Studies of Reading, 3*, 331–361.

Catts, H. W., & Kamhi, A. G. (1999). Causes of reading disabilities. In H. W. Catts & A. G. Kamhi (Eds.), *Language and reading disabilities* (pp. 95–127). Boston, MA: Allyn & Bacon.

Ciesielski, K., Courchesne, E., & Elmasian, R. (1990). Effects of focused, selective attention tasks on event-related potentials in autistic and normal individual. *Electroencephalography and Clinical Neurophysiology, 7*, 207–220.

Courchesne, E. (1991). A new model of brain and behavior development in infantile autism. *Proceedings of the Autism Society of America National Conference*, p. 25.

Cunningham, P. M. (1979). Beginning reading without readiness: Structured language experience. *Reading Horizons, 19*(3), 222–227.

Cunningham, P. M., & Allington, R. L. (2010). *Classrooms that work: They can all read and write* (5th ed.). Boston, MA: Ally & Bacon.

Cunningham, P. M., Hall, D. P., & Defee, M. (1991). Non-ability grouped, multilevel instruction: A year in a first-grade classroom. *Reading Teacher, 44*(8), 566–572.

Cunningham, P. M., Hall, D. P., & Sigmon, C. M. (1999). *The teacher's guide to the Four Blocks*. Greensboro, NC: Carson-Dellosa.

Department of Health and Human Services, Office for Civil Rights. (2006). Fact sheet: Your rights under the Section 504 of the Rehabilitation Act. Retrieved from http://www.hhs.gov/ocr/civilrights/resources/factsheets/504.pdf

Diehl, S. F., Ford, C. S., & Federico, J. (2005). The communication journey of a fully included child with an autism spectrum disorder. *Topics in Language Disorders, 25*, 375–387.

Erickson, K. A., & Koppenhaver, D. A. (2007). *Children with disabilities: Reading and writing the Four Blocks way*. Greensboro, NC: Carson-Dellosa.

Estes, A., Rivera, V., Bryan, M., Cali, P., & Dawson, G. (2011). Discrepancies between academic achievement and intellectual ability in higher-functioning school-aged children with autism spectrum disorder. *Journal of Autism and Developmental Disorders, 41*, 1044–1052.

Frith, U. (1989). Autism and "theory of mind." In C. Gillberg (Ed.), *Diagnosis and treatment of autism* (pp. 33–52). New York, NY: Plenum Press.

Frith, U., & Baron-Cohen, S. (1987). Perception in autistic children. In D. J. Cohen & A. M. Donnellan (Eds.), *Handbook of autism and pervasive developmental disorders*. New York, NY: Wiley.

Graham, S., & Hebert, M. (2010). *Writing to read: Evidence for how writing can improve reading*. New York, NY: Carnegie Corporation of New York.

Gray, C. (1994). *Comic strip conversations: Colorful illustrated interactions with student with autism and related disabilities*. Jennison, MI: Jennison Public Schools.

Happé, F. G. E. (1997). Central coherence and theory of mind in autism: Reading homographs in context. *British Journal of Developmental Psychology, 15*(1), 1–12.

Hermelin, B., & O'Connor, N. (1970). *Psychological experiments with autistic children*. London, UK: Pergamon.

Hodgden, L. A. (1999). *Solving behavior problems in autism: Improving communication with visual strategies*. Troy, MI: Quirk Roberts.

Jones, C. R. G., Happé, F., Golden, H., Marsden, A. J. S., Tregay, J., Simonoff, E., . . . Charman, T. (2009). Reading and arithmetic in adolescents with autism spectrum disorders: Peaks and dips in attainment. *Neuropsychology, 23*, 718–728.

Joseph, R. M., & Tager-Flusberg, H. (2004). The relationship of theory of mind and executive functions to symptom type and severity in children with autism. *Developmental Psychopathology, 16*(1), 137–155.

Justice, L. M. (2006a). *Clinical approaches to emergent literacy intervention*. San Diego, CA: Plural.

Justice, L. M. (2006b). Evidence-based practice, response to intervention, and the prevention of reading difficulties. *Language, Speech, and Hearing Services in Schools, 37*, 284–297.

Justice, L. M., & Pullen, P. C. (2003). Promising interventions for promoting emergent literacy skills: Three evidence-based approaches.

Topics in Early Childhood Special Education, 23, 99–113.

Koppenhaver, D. A., & Erickson, K. A. (2003). Natural emergent literacy supports for preschoolers with autism and severe communication impairments. *Topics in Language Disorders, 23,* 283–292.

Lanter, E., & Watson, L. R. (2008). Promoting literacy in students with ASD: The basics for the SLP. *Language, Speech, and Hearing Services in Schools, 39,* 33–43.

Lanter, E., Watson, L. R., Erickson, K. A., & Freeman, D. (2012). Emergent literacy in children with autism: An exploration of developmental and contextual dynamic processes. *Language, Speech, and Hearing Services in Schools, 43,* 308–324.

MacDuff, G., Krantz, P., & McClannahan, L. (1993). Teaching children with autism to use pictographic activity schedules: Maintenance and generalization of complex response chains. *Journal of Applied Behavior Analysis, 26,* 89–97.

McEvoy, R. E., Rogers, S. J., & Pennington B. F. (1993). Executive function and social communication deficits in young autistic children. *Journal of Child Psychology and Psychiatry, 34,* 563–578.

Mirenda, P. (2003). "He's not really a reader . . . ": Perspectives on supporting literacy development in individuals with autism. *Topics in Language Disorders, 23,* 271–282.

Mirenda, P., & Erickson, K. (2000). Augmentative communication and literacy. In A. M. Wetherby & B. M. Prizant (Eds.), *Autism spectrum disorders: A transactional developmental perspective* (pp. 333–367). Baltimore, MD: Paul H. Brookes.

Myles, B. S., & Southwick, J. (1999). *Asperger syndrome and difficult moments: Practical solutions for tantrums, rage and meltdowns.* Shawnee Mission, KS: Autism Asperger Publishing.

Nation, K., Clarke, P., Wright, B., & Williams, C. (2006). Patterns of reading ability in children with autism spectrum disorder. *Journal of Autism and Developmental Disabilities, 36,* 911–919.

National Early Literacy Panel. (2008). *Developing early literacy: Report of the National Early Literacy Panel.* Washington DC: National Institute for Literacy.

National Governors Association Center for Best Practices, Council of Chief State School Officers. (2010). *Common core state standards.* Washington, DC: Author.

National Institute of Child Health and Human Development. (2000). *Report of the National Reading Panel. Teaching children to read: An evidence-based assessment of the scientific research literature on reading and its implications for reading instruction.* Retrieved from https://www.nichd.nih.gov/publications/pubs/nrp/pages/smallbook.aspx

Norbury, C., & Nation, K. (2011). Understanding variability in reading comprehension in adolescents with autism spectrum disorders: Interactions with language status and decoding skill. *Scientific Studies of Reading, 15*(3), 191–210.

Notari-Syverson, A., O'Connor, R., & Vadasy, P. F. (1998). *Ladders to literacy: A preschool activity book.* Baltimore, MD: Brookes.

Nutall, G., Graesser, A., & Person, N. (2013). *Discourse classroom discourse, Cognitive perspective.* http://education.stateuniversity.com/pages/1916/Discourse.html

O'Connor, I. M., & Klein, P. D. (2004). Exploration of strategies for facilitating the reading comprehension of high-functioning students with autism spectrum disorders. *Journal of Autism and Developmental Disorders, 34*(2), 115–127.

Ozonoff, S., & McEvoy, R. E. (1994). A longitudinal study of executive function and theory of mind development in autism. *Development and Psychopathology, 6,* 415–431.

Ozonoff, S., Pennington, B. F., & Rogers, S. J. (1991). Executive function deficits in high-functioning autistic individuals: Relationship to theory of mind. *Journal of Child Psychology and Psychiatry, 32,* 1081–1105.

Paul, R. (2005). Assessing communication in autism spectrum disorders. In F. Volkmar, R. Paul, A. Klin, & D. Cohen (Eds.), *Handbook of autism and pervasive developmental disorders: Assessment, interventions, and policy* (Vol. 2, pp. 799–816). Hoboken, NJ: Wiley.

Quill, K. A. (1997). Instructional considerations for young children with autism: The rationale for visually cued instruction. *Journal of Autism and Developmental Disorders, 27*(6), 697–714.

Quill, K., & Grant, N. (1996). Visually cued instruction: Strategies to enhance communication and socialization. *Proceedings of the Autism Society of America National Conference,* Milwaukee, WI.

Randi, J., Newman, T., & Grigorenko, E. L. (2010). Teaching children with autism to read for meaning: Challenges and possibilities. *Journal of Autism and Developmental Disorders, 40,* 890–902.

Raphael, T. (1984). Teaching learners about sources of information for answering comprehension questions. *Journal of Reading, 27,* 303–311.

Savarese, D. J. (2010). Cultural commentary: Communicate with me. *Disability Studies Quarterly, 30*(1). Retrieved from http://dsq-sds.org/article/view/1051/1237

Schopler, E., Mesibov, G., & Hearsey, K. (1995). Structured teaching in the TEACCH system. In E. Schopler & G. Mesibov (Eds.), *Learning and cognition in autism.* New York, NY: Plenum Press.

Silliman, E. R., Bahr, R. H., & Peters, M. L. (2006). Spelling patterns in preadolescents with atypical language skills: Phonological, morphological, and orthographic factors. *Developmental Neuropsychology, 29,* 93–123.

Sun, L., & Wallach, G. P. (2013). Adolescent literacy: Looking beyond core language learning deficits. *Perspectives on Language Learning and Education, 20,* 57–66.

Treiman, R., & Bourassa, D. C. (2000). The development of spelling skill. *Topics in Language Disorders, 20*(3), 1–18.

Troia, G. A. (2004). Building word recognition skills through empirically validated instructional practices: Collaborative efforts of speech-language pathologists and teachers. In E. R. Silliman & L. C. Wilkinson (Eds.), *Language and literacy learning in schools* (pp. 98–129). New York, NY: Guilford Press.

Westby, C. (2002). Beyond decoding: Critical and dynamic literacy for students with dyslexia, language learning disabilities (LLD), or attention deficit-hyperactivity disorder (ADHD). In K. G. Butler & E. R. Silliman (Eds.), *Speaking, reading and writing in children with language learning disabilities: New paradigms for research and practice* (pp. 73–108). Mahwah, NJ: Erlbaum.

Westby, C., Culatta, B., Lawrence, B., & Hall-Kenyon, K. (2010). Summarizing expository texts. *Topics in Language Disorders, 30,* 275–287.

Whalon, K. J., Al Otaiba, S., & Delano, M. E. (2009). Evidence-based reading instruction for individuals with autism spectrum disorders. *Focus on Autism and Other Developmental Disabilities, 24*(1), 3–16.

Zucker, T. A., Ward, A. E., & Justice, L. M. (2009). Print referencing during read-alouds: A technique for increasing emergent readers' print knowledge. *Reading Teacher, 63,* 62–72.

7

Bringing It All Together: Application and Video Examples

Introduction

This chapter highlights four children with ASD and their families and how the strategies discussed in this book translate into real practice. Each family generously volunteered to have two graduate students from the University of Florida Department of Speech-Language and Hearing Sciences who were taking a course in autism (taught by C. Zenko) come into their homes and work with them and their children. The authors would like to thank the families for volunteering to share their children with the students and granting us permission to use the information and video footage for the purpose of this book. The authors would also like to thank the students for allowing us to showcase your assignments as a way to teach others.

The chapter provides background knowledge on each child and a brief explanation of the various videos, photos, and documents included in each case study. A table outlines the contents of each case study to act as a quick reference of what to expect on the supplemental DVD. Each case study was carefully chosen to illustrate various concepts discussed throughout this text and meant to help synthesize the essence of what the authors describe as "balanced intervention."

The DVD provides digital case studies of four children on various points of the autism spectrum. Each case study has its own menu and includes: video samples, pictures of various visual supports, and other files that the students created for each family. In some cases, the students created interactive PowerPoint books to teach certain concepts. The actual PowerPoint files are included whenever possible; however, please be sure to give proper credit to the creators if you choose to use the files in your own therapy sessions.

Case Study A: F. G.

All files and notes for Case Study A were provided by Lauren Sherman and Bonnie Needleman (2012)—graduate students at the University of Florida, Department of Speech-Language and Hearing Sciences who worked with F. G. and his family.

F. G. is a six-year-old male with a diagnosis of autism who is included in a kindergarten class with a paraprofessional. F. lives with his mom, dad, younger brother, and dog. F.'s interests include: *Shaun the Sheep*, Superman, Spiderman, Batman, painting, Legos, letters, numbers, and his LeapPad. F. G. was diagnosed at age one and one half, and according to F.'s mom, "It was 'so obvious' that F. had autism." F.'s mom listed the following signs they observed when F. was young: delayed milestones (motor and language); would sit contently in his swing chair for long periods of time; lack of eye contact; low muscle tone; breakdowns that could only be calmed by TV; trouble transitioning from one room to another; and freaking out when someone opened a door.

F. received various communication interventions from the time he was diagnosed until now. He began using PECS at 18 months and attempted to use Dynavox AAC system around the age of three but did not like it. F. spoke his first words at age four and one half, and he is hyperlexic. Today, F. communicates using verbalizations, gestures, single words, and short phrases. He relies on visual cues (more at school) and is currently receiving speech/language therapy and occupational therapy in school and ABA services for six hours per week privately.

Needleman and Sherman noted the following observations regarding F.'s ASD characteristics. F.'s unique communication features included: echolalia, abnormal prosody, and impaired language or reading comprehension. In the area of socialization, F. had: limited eye contact, more parallel play than interactive play, and a short attention span. Finally, the behavioral characteristics of ASD that the students observed were: inappropriate play, restricted interests, difficulty with transitions, and breaking things when he was left alone.

The goals the students targeted during their time with F. focused on increasing his expressive communication, answering Wh- and open-ended questions, and being able to transition to a different activity or end an activity without becoming upset.

Table 7–1 outlines the contents of all the files that illustrate Case Study A on the DVD.

Table 7–1. List and Explanation of Contents of Case Study A (on DVD)

Appendix Name	Contents
A–1: Listen to Parent's Concerns	Video of mom sharing her main concern.
A–2: Create Supports that Address Parent's Concern	Video of Lauren introducing the new home/school communication book they created to address mom's concern.
A–3: Home/School Communication Book	PowerPoint file with pictures of the home/school communication book.

Table 7–1. *continued*

Appendix Name	Contents
A–4 a & b: Timers Make Transitions Easier	Two videos showing F. using a timer to make transitions easier.
A–5: Visual Cues Make Transitions Easier	Video of F. using tri-fold visual support that outlines three steps of playing (with Legos in this video).
A–6: Tri-Fold Visual Support for Transition	Picture of the tri-fold visual support.
A–7: Using Songs with Visual Supports to Add Meaning and Repetition	Video of Bonnie singing the "hand washing song" she created to augment the hand washing visual support.
A–8: Hand Washing Visual Support	Picture of the hand washing support.
A–9 a & b: Using PPT Books to Address IEP Goals—Collaborate with All Therapists to Work on Goals	Two videos of Lauren and Bonnie showing F. the PowerPoint books they made for him.
A–10 a & b: PowerPoint Books for Teaching: (a) Wh-Questions; (b) Categorization	Actual PowerPoint book files.
A–11: Visual Supports Help F. Answer Open-Ended Questions	Video showing F. using a visual choice board to pick where he wants to go.

Case Study B: A. H.

All files and notes for Case Study B were provided by Molly Wells Vogeli and Shannon Filipponi (2010), Maria Burnes and Lauren McElhinney (2012)—graduate students at the University of Florida, Department of Speech-Language and Hearing Sciences who worked with A. H. and her family.

A. H. is a nine-year-old female with autism who is included in a fourth-grade class at a private school. She lives with her mom, dad, younger brother, and sister. A.'s interests include: Pixie Hollow, fairies, and Lalaloopsy. A.'s mom describes her as advanced for her age prior to age two and then began to regress. She was diagnosed with PDD-NOS at age two and began occupational and speech/language therapy. At age four, she was reevaluated and received an autism diagnosis. A. is on a gluten- and casein-free diet, and receives B-12 shots. A.'s strengths include: reading, math, using scripts, following schedules, memory, and an outgoing personality. Her weaknesses are: focus and attention, staying on task, joining a group of peers, eye contact, reading comprehension, retelling narratives, following conversational rules (e.g., looking at or facing a person when talking to them), awareness of social appropriateness, and active listening.

A. communicates by speaking and has an extensive vocabulary. Burnes and McElhinney described A.'s communication, sensory processing, and social interaction characteristics that they observed that are consistent with her autism diagnosis. A.'s communication includes unusual, "commercial-like" prosody when she is telling a story or echoing phrases from TV shows, occasional dysfluencies, and decreased eye contact. Her sensory processing differences include: frequent chewing on objects (she uses "Chewelry," jewelry she can chew on), hypotonicity, low energy, and hypersensitivity to the noise and crowd during recess. Socially, A. has difficulty: understanding personal space and knowing the hidden rules or pragmatic language skills that most children know innately, but she is very social and likes to interact with people.

Table 7–2. List and Explanation of Contents of Case Study B (on DVD)

Appendix Name	Contents
B–1: The Art of Conversation	Video of Molly and Shannon having a conversation with A. What do you notice about A.'s conversational/pragmatic skills?
B–2: Listening and Reading Comprehension	Video showing Molly and Shannon working on listening and reading comprehension skills. What supports does A. need to be successful?
B–3: Working on Eye Contact in a Fun, Natural Context	Video of A. playing Candyland with her brother, Molly, and Shannon. The students established a rule that A. had to look at Shannon and ask for a card each turn.
B–4: Reading Comprehension: Vocabulary and Prediction	Video of A. reading a Curious George book on the computer. The students use the book to teach the word "spotted" and to have A. predict what will happen next.
B–5: Figurative Language	Video of A. reading Peter Pan and the opportunity came up to teach the expression, "licking his chops."
B–6: Using a Graphic Organizer to Retell a Story	Video of A. working on retelling a story with the help of a graphic organizer. She struggles with some of the open-ended questions. What scaffolds do the students use to help her?
B–7: Teaching the Meaning of Idioms	PowerPoint book created by Maria Burnes to teach A. about idioms.
B–8: Using Interests and Video Modeling to Teach Inferencing	PowerPoint book created by Lauren McElhinney using A.'s interest in Lalaloopsy to teach inferencing skills. The book uses links to YouTube videos of Lalaloopsy for A. to watch and then answer questions about the video (example of how to use video modeling).

The goals the students targeted while working with A. were: improving eye contact, listening comprehension, reading comprehension, inferencing, and understanding figurative language.

Table 7–2 outlines the contents of all the files that illustrate Case Study B on the DVD.

Case Study C: C. S.

All files and notes for Case Study C were provided by Jennifer Boyd and Vanessa Frieler (2012)—graduate students at the University of Florida, Department of Speech-Language and Hearing Sciences who worked with C. S. and his family.

C. S. is a 12-year-old boy with Asperger syndrome (AS) who is included in the seventh grade with a paraprofessional. C. was diagnosed with AS at age four and one half but had obvious sensory issues around age two that included extreme reactions to loud noises that involved him crawling underneath heavy objects to escape the noise. He also has sensory integration dysfunction and attention deficit hyperactivity disorder diagnoses. He lives with his mom, dad, older sister, dog, and guinea pig. C.'s interests include: Star Wars, Power Rangers, Club Penguin, playing games on the computer, and animals. His strengths include memory and computer skills. C.'s weaknesses are: maintaining control of his emotions, regulating his actions when upset, reading social cues, and interacting with same-age peers.

Boyd and Frieler described the characteristics associated with ASD that they observed when working with C. In the social interaction domain, C. had limited eye contact (improving), reduced empathy, "acts out" or is dramatic, emotional outbursts when upset, extreme reactions to minor situations, "righteous thinker," and difficulty sharing with others. C. communicated verbally and had a very advanced expressive vocabulary; however, he frequently interrupted, talked incessantly about interests, interpreted things literally, talked to himself, and used different voices when he was upset. The restricted or repetitive behaviors observed included: intense preoccupation with certain things, perseveration on topics, very routine-oriented, and his body movements became rigid, accelerated, and repetitive when he was upset. Finally, C.'s sensory concerns were illustrated by: being agitated by loud noises (alarms, lightning, fire drills), disliked certain clothing textures (wet clothes), avoided being touched when emotions were elevated, and was a very picky eater.

Table 7–3. List and Explanation of Contents of Case Study C (on DVD)

Appendix Name	Contents
C–1: Texting and Calling New Friends	A story created by Jennifer Boyd to teach C. about the hidden rules of not calling or texting a new friend too much.
C–2: Dating Space	A story created to teach C. that he needs to give his sister space when she is out on a date (PPT file).
C–3 a: Substitute Survival Guide—Substitute's Copy **b:** Substitute Survival Guide—Student Copy **c:** Substitute Survival Guide—Blank Template	The Substitute Survival Guide was a visual support that C. helped the students make to help him make it through the day when there was a substitute. It has two parts. **a:** Is the explanation of what Asperger syndrome is, how it affects C., and things that work for C. This part is given to the substitute. **b:** Is a visual support for the student (C.) to keep to remind him or her of strategies to use to stay calm. **c:** Is just a blank template of Part A (the substitute's copy) for you to use with your own students.
C–4: C.'s perspective—Substitute Survival Guide—Substitute Copy	A video of C. explaining what the substitute survival guide is and why it works to give to substitutes.
C–5: C.'s perspective- Substitute Survival Guide- His Copy	A video of C. explaining how he uses his part of the Substitute Survival Guide.
C–6: Group Work Can Be Fun	A story for C. to help him be more successful during group work (in PowerPoint book format).
C–7: Star Wars 5-Point Scale	A video of C. explaining a 5-Point Scale* that a graduate student created for him using his interest in Star Wars to help depict the different levels of frustration and strategies he can do for each level.
C–8: Reducing Fractions	An interactive, personalized PowerPoint book that incorporated C.'s interests while teaching him a math concept he found difficult.
C–9: *Just Because*—A Poem Written by C. This Year	A poem that C. wrote for his writing class that demonstrates his perspective on having ASD.

*Buron, K. D., & Curtis, M. B. (2012). *The incredible 5-point scale: The significantly improved and expanded second edition: Assisting students in understanding social interactions and controlling their emotional responses.* Overland Park, KS: Autism Asperger Publishing Company.

The students addressed concerns that C. and his family expressed at both home and school. At home, C. was having trouble respecting his sister's privacy. He also needed guidance about the hidden rules of texting new friends. For school, the students targeted three main issues: (1) working successfully in groups; (2) understanding fractions; and (3) coping when there was a substitute teacher.

Table 7–3 outlines the contents of all the files that illustrate Case Study C on the DVD.

Case Study D: M. S.

All files and notes for Case Study D were provided by Heather Caseres and Desiree Williams (2012)—graduate students at the University of Florida, Department of Speech-Language and Hearing Sciences who worked with M. S. and his family.

M. S. is a 13-year-old boy with autism who is included in regular education classes for most of the day, except for reading and math when he is in ESE classes. M. had a significant medical history prior to his autism diagnosis. When he was 15 months old, he was not meeting his motor milestones, and the family suspected he might have cerebral palsy. They saw a neurologist who ordered an MRI that revealed a brain tumor in his cerebellum, which was treated with chemotherapy. M. received early intervention services starting with physical therapy (at 18 months), speech/language therapy (at age two), occupational therapy (at age three), and applied behavior analysis. He did not receive his autism diagnosis until he turned four. M. lives with his mom, dad, and older sister. His interests include: computer, iPad, trains, animals, playing soccer, riding his bike, and enjoying sweets. M.'s strengths are: being polite, great memory, and a visual learner. His main weakness is making friends.

Caseres and Williams described the behaviors they observed in the communication, socialization, and restricted or repetitive behavior domains consistent with an autism diagnosis. M.'s unique communication characteristics included: echolalia (immediate), stuttering, unusual prosody, speech and language errors, perseverative phrases, breathy voice, and atypical pitch range. M.'s socialization differences were: spontaneous or inappropriate laughter, not assertive in stating what he wants, people-pleaser, and anxiety during unfamiliar circumstances. Finally, the following restricted or repetitive behaviors were observed: arm flapping, facial tics, body posturing (variety), rocking, and vocalizations.

The students addressed concerns that M. and his family expressed during the interview process. M.'s mom shared that M. does not like it when new people come over to the house. He gets extremely agitated and repeatedly asks when they are leaving. Heather and Desiree experienced this first-hand and used their experience to create a visual support for M. that outlines the following "unknowns:" who, when, and where before a new person comes over. Another issue the family expressed is being able to go out to dinner and enjoy their time in the restaurant together. M. has trouble keeping his hands and body still and often distracts his family and others in the restaurant. Making mistakes and then fixing

Table 7–4. List and Explanation of Contents of Case Study D (on DVD)

Appendix Name	Contents
D–1: OK Go Home	Video of M. during the students' first visit to his home. He does not like new people in his house and is agitated. His involuntary motor movements get worse when he is stressed.
D–2: Who When Where Support	Picture of the temporal visual support that Desiree made to help reduce M.'s anxiety about new people coming over to his house and to use in any other situation to help plan out what to expect.
D–3: Who When Where Introduction	Video of Desiree explaining the support to M. and his mom and brainstorm ideas of when they can use the support.
D–4: Who When Where Explanation	Video of Desiree showing M. how to use his new support and practicing filling it out.
D–5: Who When Where Practice	Video of M. using the support to help prepare him for a new person coming to his house.
D–6: Going to Dinner Social Story	Story that Heather wrote for M. to help teach and remind him what is expected of him when the family goes out to dinner using a PowerPoint book format.
D–7: Going to Dinner Introduction	Video of Heather showing M. the Going to Dinner PowerPoint and following up with comprehension check questions.
D–8: Making Mistakes Social Story	Story that Desiree made for M. to explain that everyone makes mistakes, and it is OK. M. does not like it when he makes mistakes.
D–9: Making Mistakes Presentation	Video of Desiree reading the social story with M. and adding in comprehension questions along the way.
D–10: Recognizing Emotions	An interactive PowerPoint book that Desiree created to teach M. about recognizing emotions.
D–11: Emotion Practice	A video of M. trying to guess what emotion Desiree is feeling based on her facial expression and body language. They had just read the PowerPoint book and are now following up with a little practice.
D–12: Making Change ($)	An interactive PowerPoint book that Heather created to teach M. about the monetary concept of change.
D–13: Making Change—A Multisensory Approach	Video of Heather showing M. the PowerPoint book about making change. The book is interactive, and she has real money on the table to have hands-on practice with what is on the screen.

the mistakes was another area M. had trouble doing, so Desiree created an informational story about making mistakes. Understanding emotions and learning how to make change (money) were the last two topics the students went over with M.

Table 7–4 outlines the contents of all the files that illustrate Case Study D on the DVD.

Summary

As illustrated by the video and other support files on the DVD, the case examples demonstrate the vast array of strengths and difficulties that can be seen in individuals on the autism spectrum. This variability makes working with children with ASD both exciting and challenging. Although each of the four cases is uniquely different, we hope the reader can see the core characteristics of ASD that unite each child. Chapters 1 through 6 give the reader the foundational knowledge about the core cognitive and social communication challenges associated with a diagnosis of ASD. The current chapter provides an opportunity to put this knowledge into practice in similar yet different ways, in addition to practice pairing this information with the family's desires, culture, and so forth. The reader can see the pieces of the puzzle come together in each of the four cases, as the clinicians and caregivers sought to create a balanced intervention for each child that took into account the functional needs of the child at home, in the community, and at school.

Index

Note: Page numbers in **bold** reference non-text material.

C

W